MW01603020

Uncomplicated Tuscan Cooking

Cucina Semplice Toscana

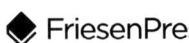 FriesenPress

Suite 300 - 990 Fort St
Victoria, BC, Canada, V8V 3K2
www.friesenpress.com

Copyright © 2016 by Arcadia's Kitchen
First Edition — 2016

All rights reserved.

No part of this publication may be reproduced in any form, or
by any means, electronic or mechanical, including photocopying,
recording, or any information browsing, storage, or retrieval
system, without permission in writing from FriesenPress.

ISBN
978-1-4602-7664-8 (Hardcover)
978-1-4602-5647-3 (Paperback)
978-1-4602-5648-0 (eBook)

1. Cooking, Regional & Ethnic, Italian

Distributed to the trade by The Ingram Book Company

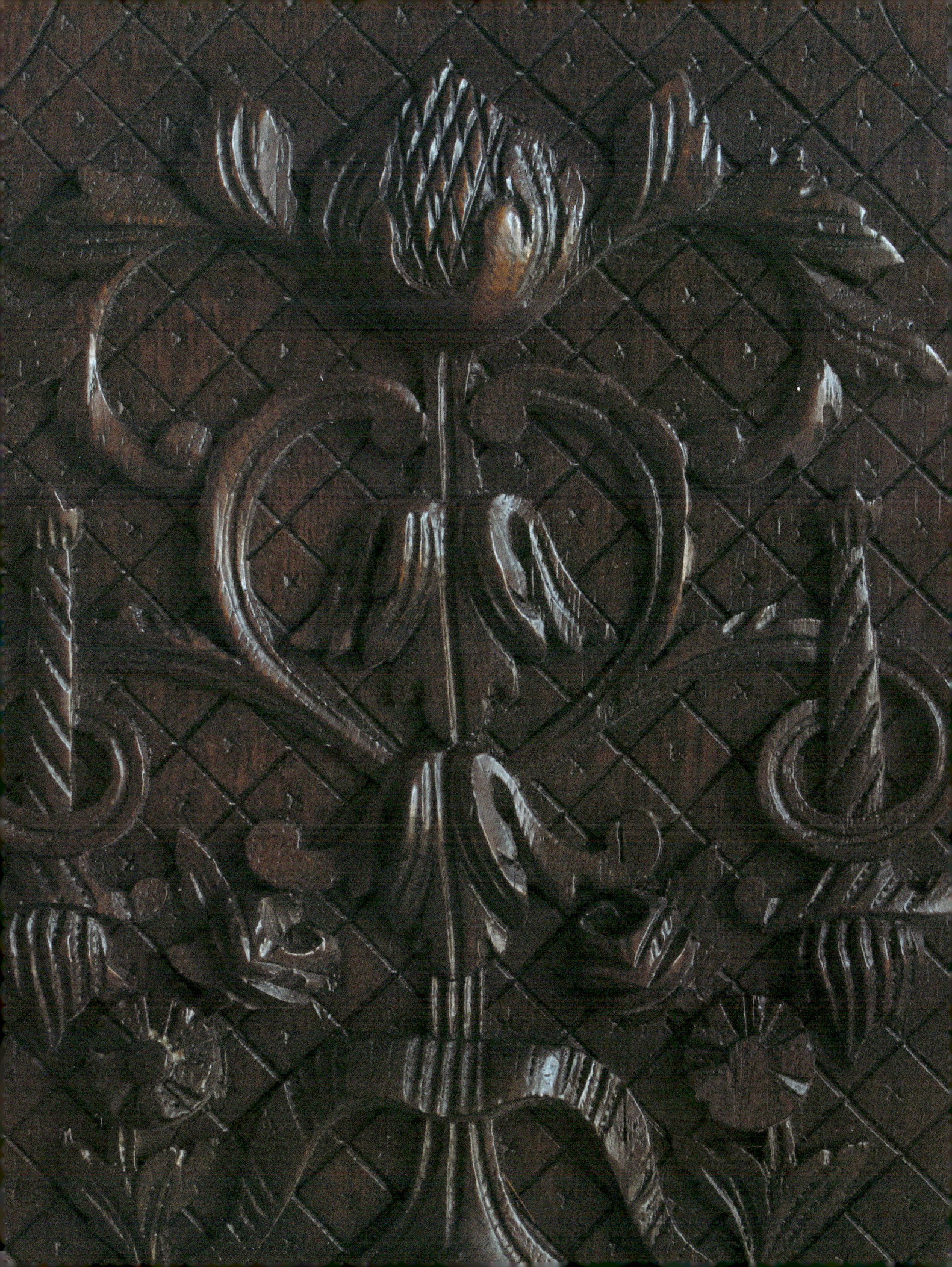

Uncomplicated Tuscan Cooking

Cucina Semplice Toscana

by

Luis Somoza & Robert Gray

To all the strong women in our lives—grandmothers, mothers, aunts—who made us who we are today and showed us that cooking is love.

Si deve mangiar per vivere,
non vivere per mangiare!

You should eat to live, not live to eat!

CONTENTS

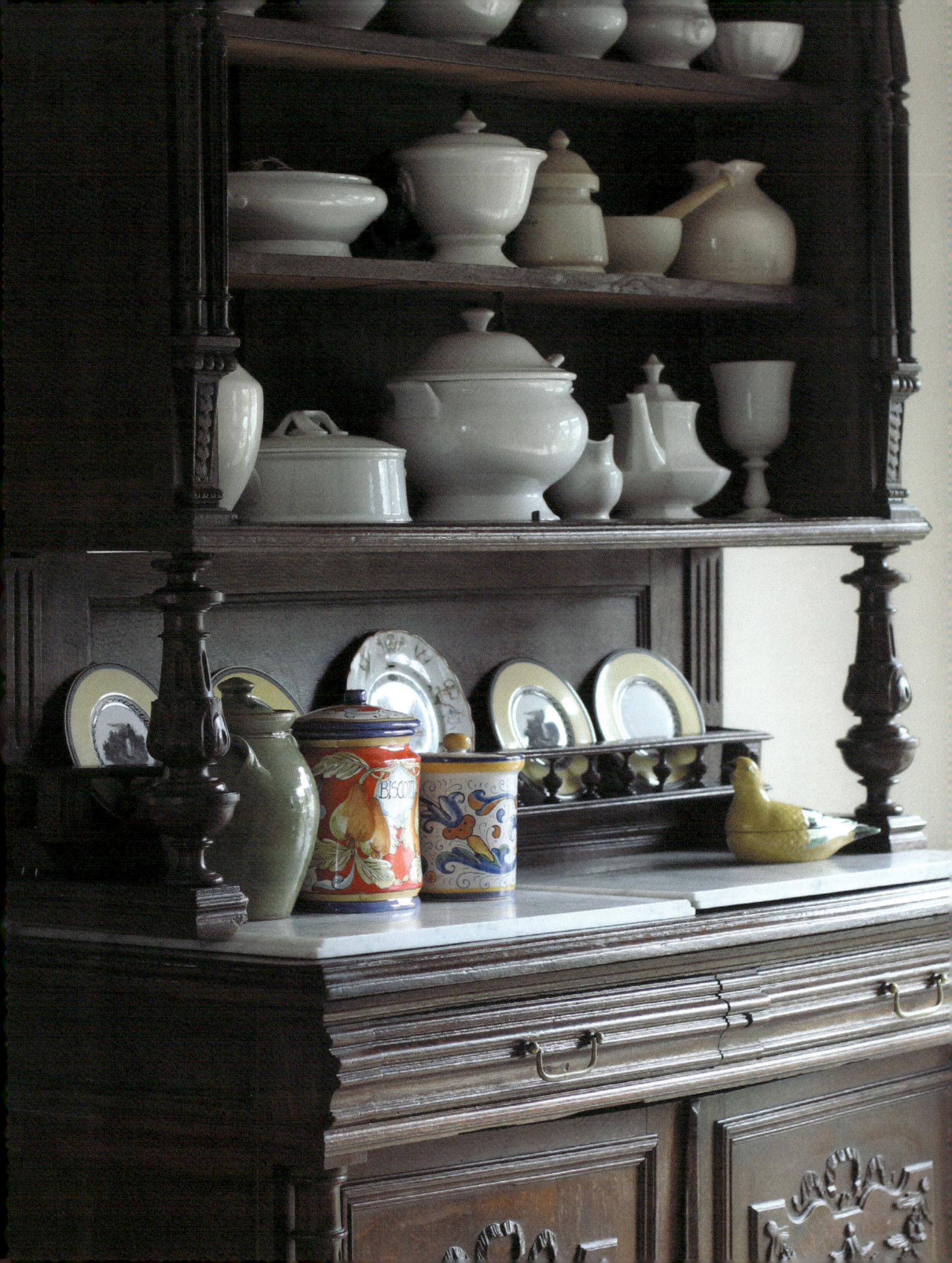

PREFACE

Most of the recipes in this book can be prepared as they are in Italy: with freshness and simplicity, and without an endless list of ingredients that you may never use again.

Fresh herbs like basil, rosemary, and sage, along with sea salt and extra virgin olive oil, prevail throughout most of the recipes— including desserts!—achieving the innate and uncomplicated way of Italian home cooking

The techniques and recipes are handed down by the grand dames in my family, and two venerable nonnas, in the hills of Florence and Fiesole and on the quaint island of Torcello in Venice.

Both groups of women had this in common: a passion for cooking and the lack of measurements written for recipes. They never wrote them down since they knew what they were doing; their simple measurements were *al occhio* (by the eye), *un pugno* (a handful), *un pizzico* (a pinch of), and *al ditto* (by the finger). What I've shared in this book comes from my own memories.

From times of abundance and scarcity, this book is an ode to the uncomplicated and resourceful way of Italian cooking.

My passion for cooking has been ingrained in me since early childhood by observing the way my family cooked. This passion later evolved from a range of abundance, need,

and hunger, and then again from the bounty of foods only the United States and Italy could offer.

During my childhood, we experienced times of plenitude, and enjoyed the diversity of both local and international foods as well as family recipes handed down from generation to generation. Some of those recipes seemed like grandiose productions that required a small army of women to create. The grains, vegetables, and fruits would arrive early in the morning, just as I was on my way to school; when I returned for lunch, they would be magically transformed into the most delicious dishes featuring traditional flavors dictated by the season and festivities, and mastered through classic techniques.

There was direct contact with the land since there were few (if any) middlemen. Some of the fowl became my pets for a brief time; I fed them and made warm little nests for them to spend the night. The following day I was told the bird flew home—not exactly true; the bird was actually lunch. Many birds followed that same path throughout those early years.

There was the milk woman, in her beautiful peasant attire, who would dutifully arrive at 8:00 a.m. with her precious cargo of fresh butter and milk, and the occasional fresh ears of corn from her own garden in the countryside. Sometimes there was a gift for me in one of her baskets: homemade sweet, candied slices of pumpkin or a chunk of the most beautiful deep red clay I had ever seen, which I used for making clay models.

My maternal grandmother, Arcadia, who had owned restaurants in her younger years, first ran the kitchen. Her foods were a combination of the old and new lands. There were no measurements to her recipes, just a handful, a pinch, and some other secrets that gave her dishes that special twist.

I remember the big table in the middle of the kitchen; it always seemed to be the center of life in that large house. I used to hide underneath the table to keep from the organized chaos, hot pots, and knives, and from there would watch the whole cooking scene take place. That space under the table felt like my own little balcony from which I would watch that entire spectacle unfold.

That kitchen and table were the places where I regularly sought solace and companionship from an isolated and sheltered life. My grandmother would usually give me a taste, a morsel of her creations, in response to my persistent pulling on her apron.

When my grandmother passed away, the responsibility of the kitchen passed to my mother. Already a great cook in her own right, she still sought new cuisines, techniques, and ingredients. I was her companion at her cooking classes, and perhaps the only kid among all those women. But soon those years of abundance would come to a halt in a very drastic manner. Political turmoil and life-changing events brought an end to the stillness and quiet of an earlier time to which we could never return.

Forced to face a new reality in a land that was trying to pull itself from almost-similar circumstances of the land we left, we arrived in post-Franco Spain and learned to make do with the little we could get or whatever we could grow in the center court garden. Meat was scarce, and if something was available, it was usually not of the best quality.

My early fascination was Italian cuisine, particularly Tuscan cuisine, which I felt in tune with on a more personal level. Tuscan cooking is sober and presents simple tastes prepared with expertise and mastery. The simplicity of the dishes is rooted in a deep cultural history of poverty and misery, the *cucina povera*. For centuries, the difficult conditions of life imposed poor, inexpensive food upon the Tuscan population.

I was fascinated by other famous chefs who were the portals to their respective cuisines— Julia Child, Prosper Montagne, and Urbain Dubois, among others—but the uncomplicated way of Italian cooking is what I really fell in love with.

Italian food magazines and Italian cookbooks were my constant companions; I could only dream of those wonderful and delicious looking dishes I saw in pictures. My only option was to mimic those recipes with what we had on hand, sometimes just to try to mask the unpleasant reality when the only thing we had to eat were the less desirable cut of meats or parts of the animal.

When I finally realized my dream of learning how to cook Italian, the real Italian way of cooking became a reality when I went into total immersion with a venerable Tuscan nonna, la Signora Maria, at her house in the town of Fiesole, up on the hills above Florence. Fiesole is the Florentine "hill station", the location to which the Florentine aristocracy retired when Florence became insufferably hot in mid-summer. Not surprisingly, the Etruscans built their city at Fiesole and not down in the humid Arno River valley below.

Daily trips to the market early in the morning were the norm, picking up the best produce sold at the stalls of the open air market, fresh meats at the local butcher, and making constant stops to say hello to the owners of the various shops and stores.

Although la Signora Maria barely spoke English and I barely spoke Italian, cooking was still simple and proved to be our common language. Disapproving looks were given every time I would not follow directions. Cooking was seasonal, fresh, and uncomplicated.

When the meal was served, she would always say, *Si deve mangiar per vivere, non vivere per mangiare!* which means, "You should eat to live, not live to eat!"

—Luis Somoza

CONDIMENTS

Condimenti

Most restaurant cooks make everything from scratch: six different kinds of stock, sauces, several different cut of meats—you name it, they will make it and have it all ready.

That's all fantastic when you have an army of pros working around the clock. But for the rest of us with long hours spent in our day jobs, long commutes to and from suburbia, and reality TV addictions, it's not realistic. So here we give you three choices: the traditional pestle, the food processor, and the most convenient, good-quality store-bought pesto.

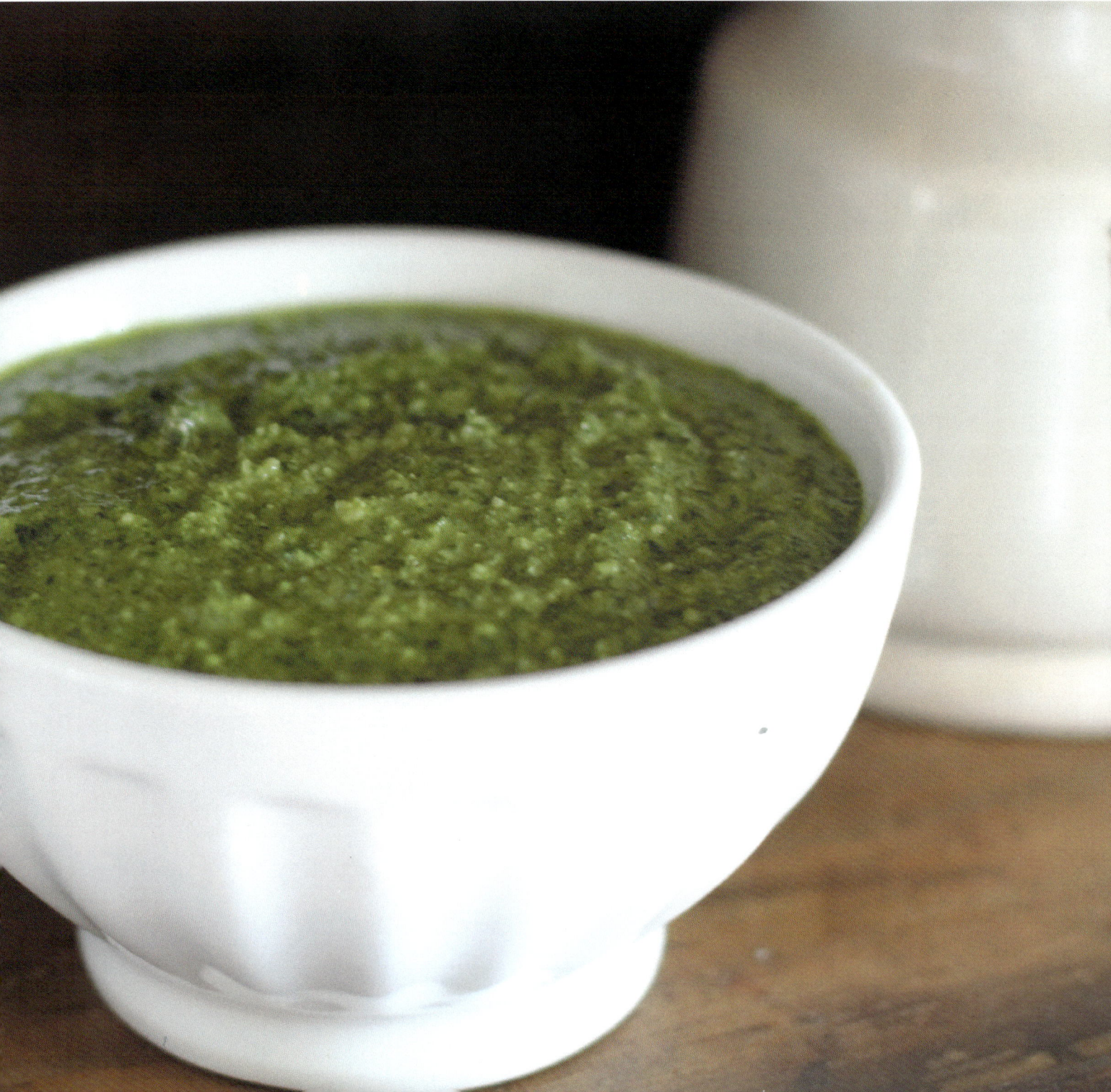

PESTO

Makes approximately 1½ cups

Pesto is one of the most recognizable and timeless symbols of Italian cuisine. Pesto recipes dating back to the 1800s didn't necessarily use basil as the main ingredient, using only a couple of leaves and some garlic. This mix was popular among the Ligurian seamen; they thought it would help ward off sickness during long sea voyages.

Pesto can refer to almost any mix of herbs that are pounded together and put over pasta. This includes arugula, parsley, mint, and tarragon, among others. In Sicily, for example, *pesto rosso* uses tomato and almonds.

Ingredients

Large handful fresh basil leaves

1 clove garlic

4½ ounces pine nuts

Extra virgin olive oil

4½ ounces hard Parmesan or Pecorino cheese, freshly grated

Pestle and mortar method:

Put the basil, garlic, and pine nuts into a pestle and mortar and crush until it is reduced to a paste.

Add enough olive oil to give a consistency you like and mix in the cheese.

Transfer to a clean dish and either use immediately or place an airtight container.

Cover in a layer of olive oil, place in the refrigerator until ready to use.

Food processor method:

Insert the chopping blade into the work bowl of the food processor.

With the machine running, drop the cheese and garlic through the feed tube to process until finely chopped, about 30 seconds. Add the nuts and pulse to chop, about five to six times. Add the basil and, using 10 to 15 long pulses, chop. Scrape the bowl and add the salt. With the machine running, add the olive oil in a slow, steady stream through the feed tube, processing until combined and an emulsion is formed, about one minute. Scrape down the sides of the work bowl.

Cover in a layer of olive oil and place in the refrigerator until ready to use.

Store bought:

Pick a good-quality pesto; be mindful of the amount of salt when adding it to your recipes as the jarred sauce already has a good amount.

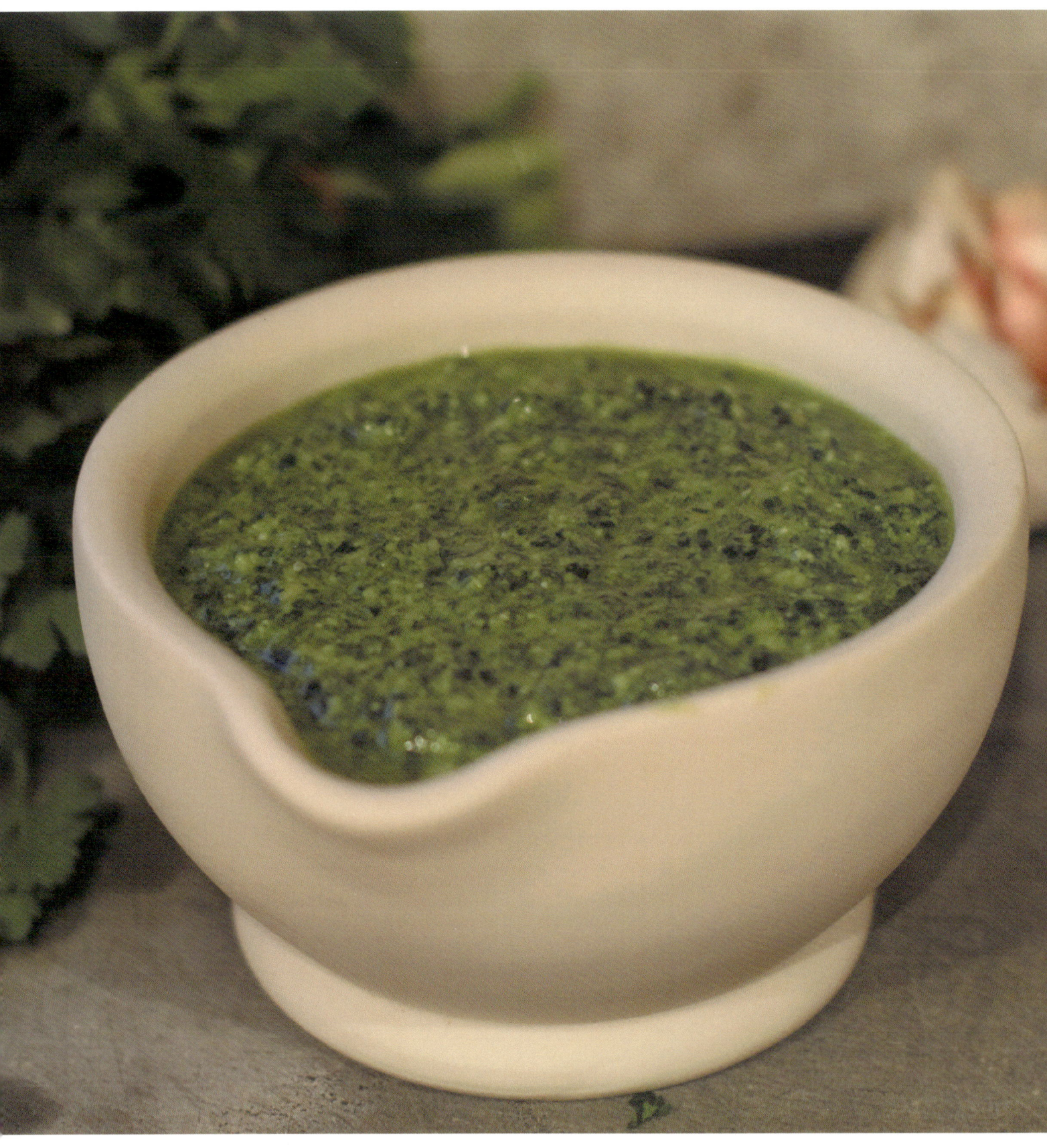

PARSLEY PESTO
Pesto di Prezzemolo

Makes approximately 1½ cups

If you think that Italian pesto is only made with basil, you're missing out on some other incredible pesto sauces. Sienese cuisine is enjoyed for the intense flavors gifted by herbs. Parsley combined with walnuts is the perfect base for pesto and a delicious addition to vegetables such as string beans and grilled fish.

Ingredients

2 cups chopped parsley

1 cup walnuts, shelled

½ cup grated parmesan cheese

3 garlic cloves, peeled and chopped

½ cup extra olive oil

Sea salt

Put the parsley, walnuts, cheese and garlic in a food processor and pulse for a few seconds to combine. Drizzle in the olive oil while the machine is running just long enough to incorporate the oil, about 20–30 seconds.

Season with sea salt, if necessary.

Use immediately or refrigerate in a sealed container until ready to use.

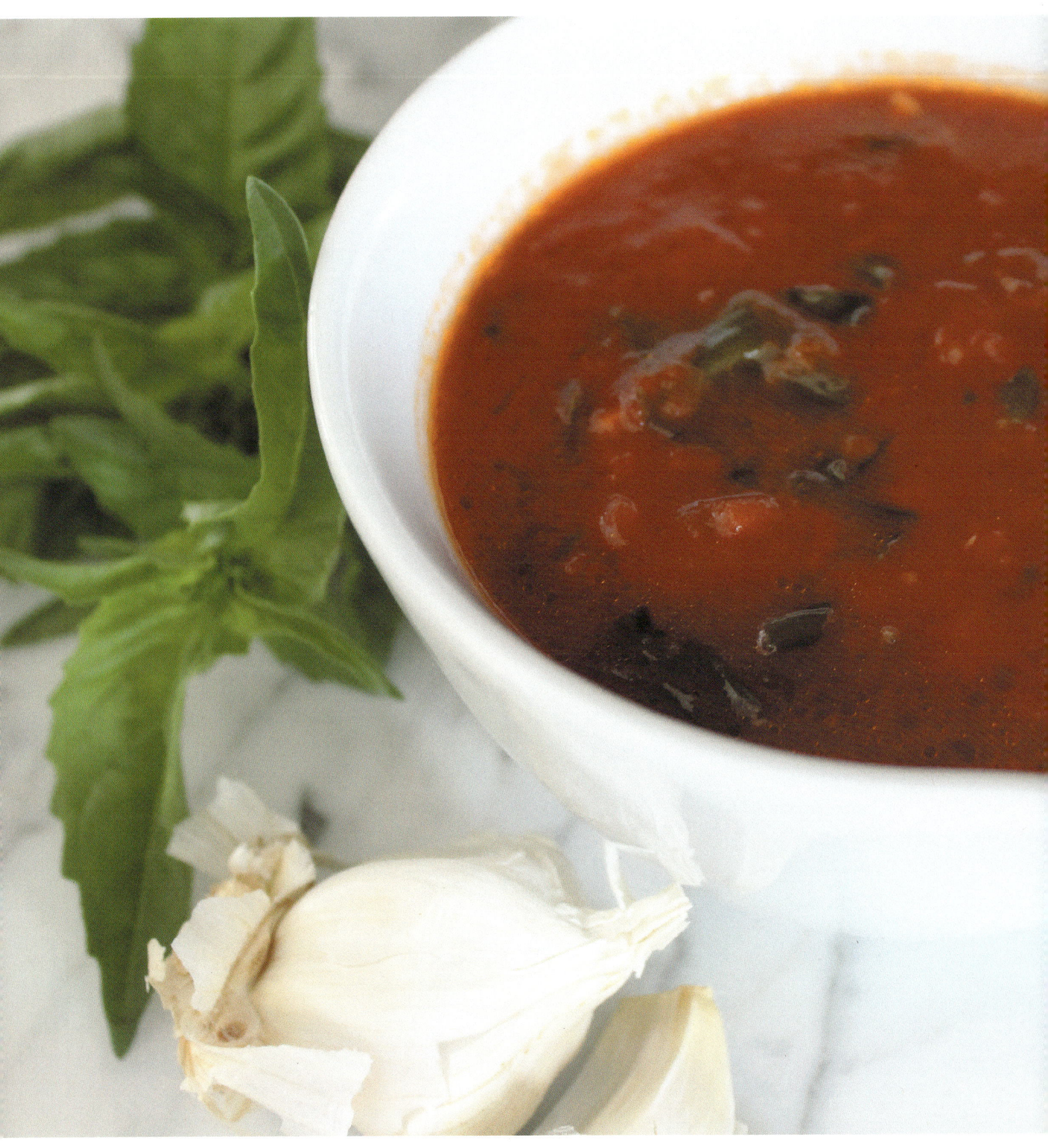

QUICK TOMATO SAUCE WITH FRESH BASIL

Salsa di Pomodoro Facile

Makes approximately 4 cups

When I first arrived in Fiesole (a town north of Florence) to live and learn to cook with a wonderful sweet nonna, I was caught by surprise at how quickly Nonna Maria could make this tomato sauce. I was expecting a pot of sauce cooking for hours; instead, it took 15 minutes at the most. The result was a fresh, bright, and delicious sauce, better than any jarred or canned.

Ingredients

4 tablespoons olive oil

3 garlic cloves, finely chopped

Peperoncini (red pepper flakes) to taste

1 (26 ounces) can of crushed Italian tomatoes

1 small bunch of fresh basil, chopped (approximately one cup)

1 cup water

Sea salt

In a large saucepan, heat the olive oil over medium heat. Add the garlic and pepperoncino and cook until the garlic releases its aroma; do not let the garlic turn brown.

Add the tomatoes in their juice, along with the basil and a cup of water. Season with salt, stir, and cook uncovered for 15 minutes.

Serve over pasta or as an addition to other recipes.

APPETIZERS

Antipasti

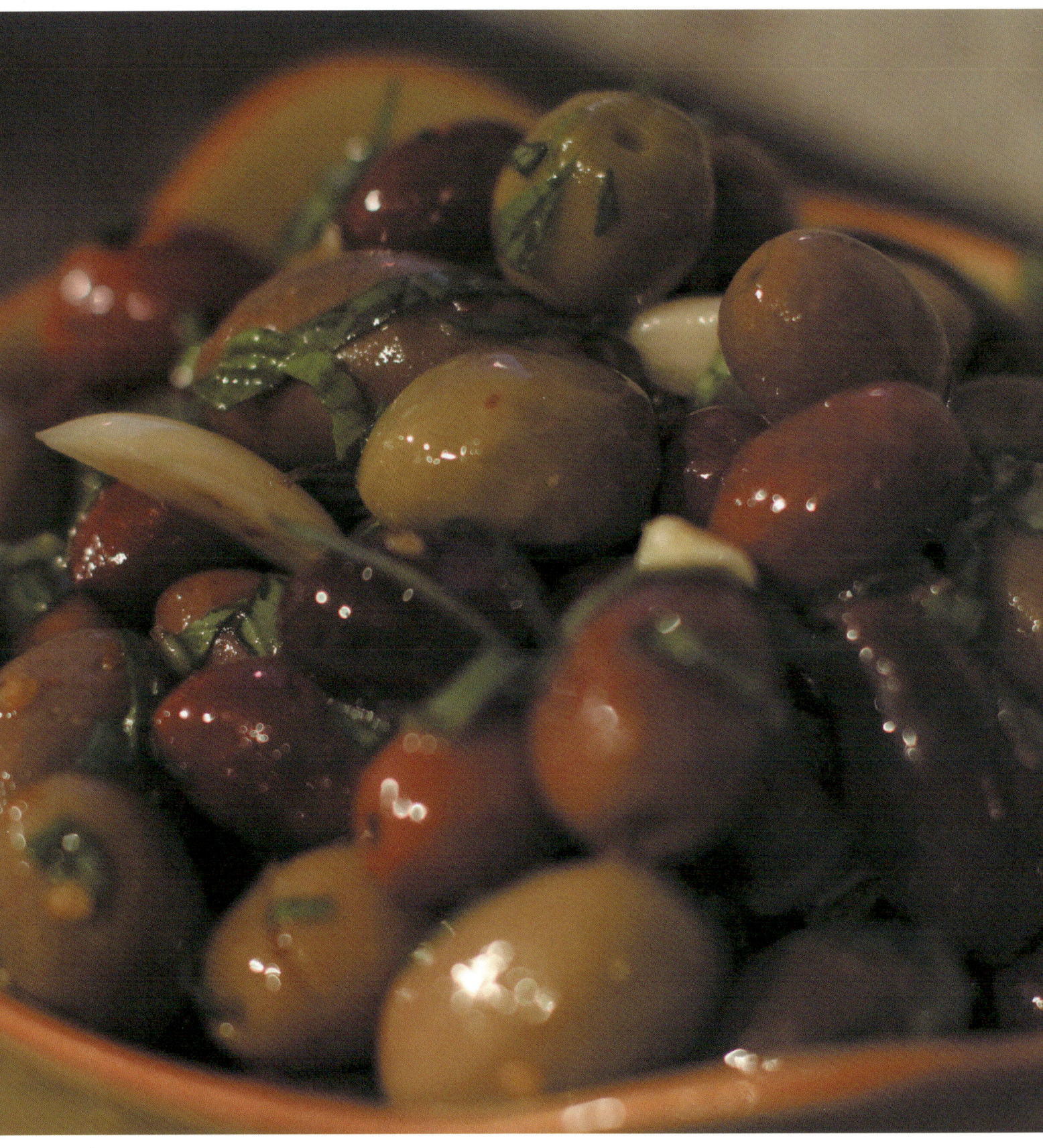

MARINATED OLIVES WITH FRESH BASIL, GARLIC & ROSEMARY

Olive in Olio Aromatizzato

Serves 4–6

Olives are a very popular and inexpensive snack and antipasto in Italy. These olives are flavored with basic ingredients such as fresh basil, rosemary, garlic and some red pepper flakes to add a level of spiciness. Mix different types of olives from the olives bar, green and black, for they all add a different layer of flavor and consistency to this simple appetizer. Do not use olives from a can, as they lack flavor and body. You can make this recipe your own by using the ingredients you have at hand and to your own taste. Try our version below and make adjustments as you like.

Ingredients

1 pound olives

4 garlic cloves, lightly crushed

10–12 large fresh basil leaves, finely chopped

1 small spring fresh rosemary, finely chopped

Peperoncini (red pepper flakes) to taste

2 tablespoons extra virgin olive oil

Mix all ingredients together in a large bowl. Chill in the refrigerator for a few hours to let the flavors mingle.

Serve at room temperature as an appetizer or accompaniment to cocktails.

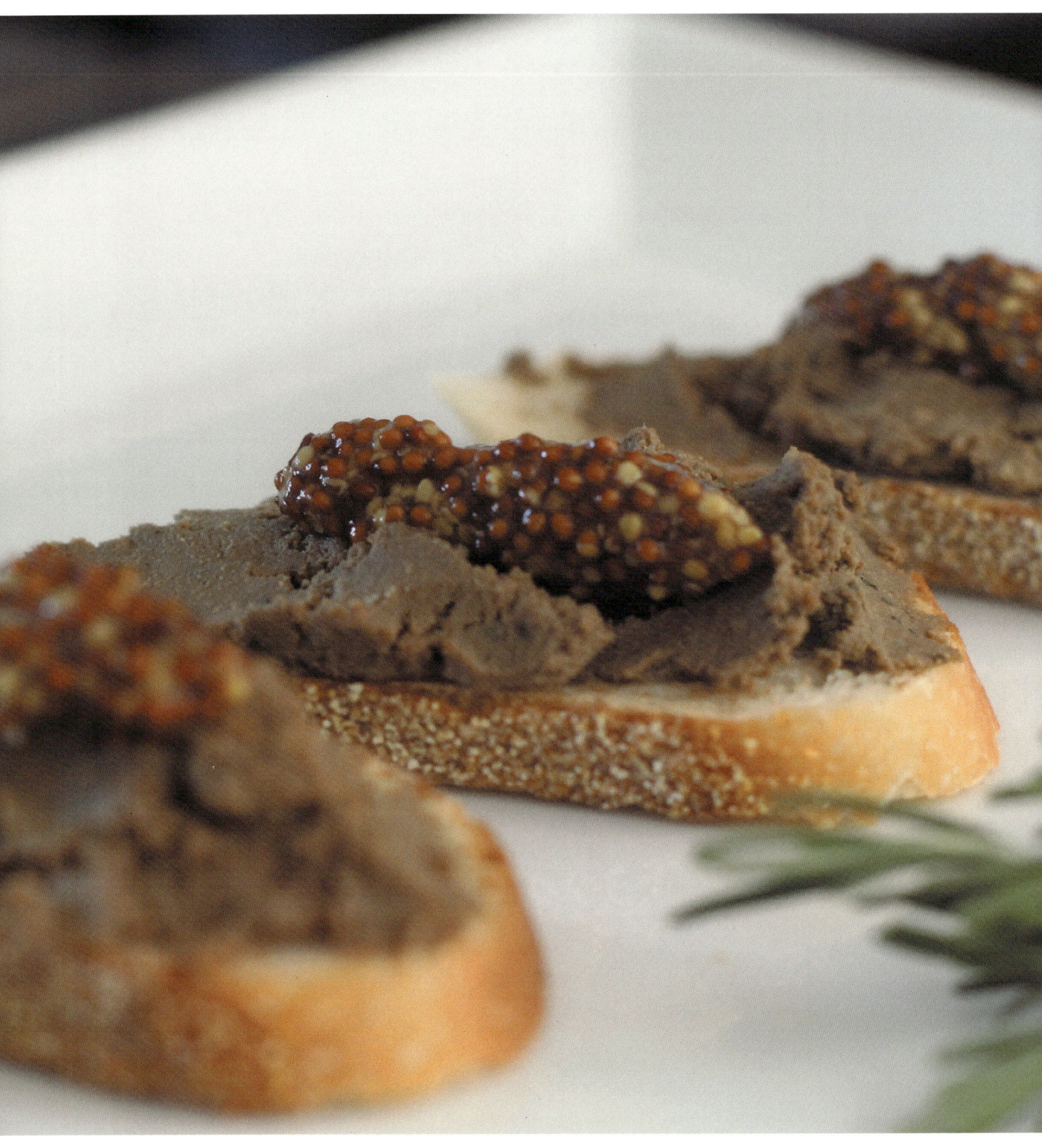

CHICKEN LIVER CROSTINI WITH COUNTRY STYLE MUSTARD

Crostini di Fegato di Pollo con Mostarda

Serves 4–5

This is a simple, classic Florentine chicken-liver pâté, which can be prepared in a coarse or smooth style. To make the rustic recipe more elegant and to introduce an additional layer of flavor, add a small amount of country-style Dijon mustard. The brine flavor of the mustard creates a nice contrast with the sweetness of the liver.

Liver has an intrinsic flavor and high fat content, so it requires a fully flavored wine; a medium bodied Pinot Noir or red Burgundy are a a good match to the rich flavors in this appetizer.

Ingredients

1/4 cup extra virgin olive oil

1 white onion, finely chopped

1 rosemary sprig, finely chopped

2 sage sprigs, finely chopped

1 pound chicken livers, trimmed and chopped

1/4 cup white wine

1½ cup chicken stock

Sea salt and freshly ground pepper

Thin slices of Tuscan bread or baguette, thinly sliced and toasted

---

Trim the chicken livers of any tough fibrous tissue and veins.

In a frying pan or skillet, sauté the onion in the olive oil until light brown. Add the chopped rosemary and sage and cook for a few minutes over medium heat, stirring frequently, until the herbs start to release their aroma. Add the chicken livers to the onion mixture and cook until it starts to brown.

Add the wine and continue cooking until the alcohol has evaporated. Add the chicken stock, keeping a small amount aside (around ½ cup) to add during the final phase of cooking. Season with salt and pepper.

Cook over low heat, stirring occasionally for a few minutes. Keep the mixture from drying out by carefully adding the reserved amount of chicken stock or water.

Remove the pan from the heat and let it cool enough to handle. Purée mixture in a food processor until very smooth.

Spoon the liver mixture over the toasted bread and top with mustard.

Serve immediately or refrigerate for later use.

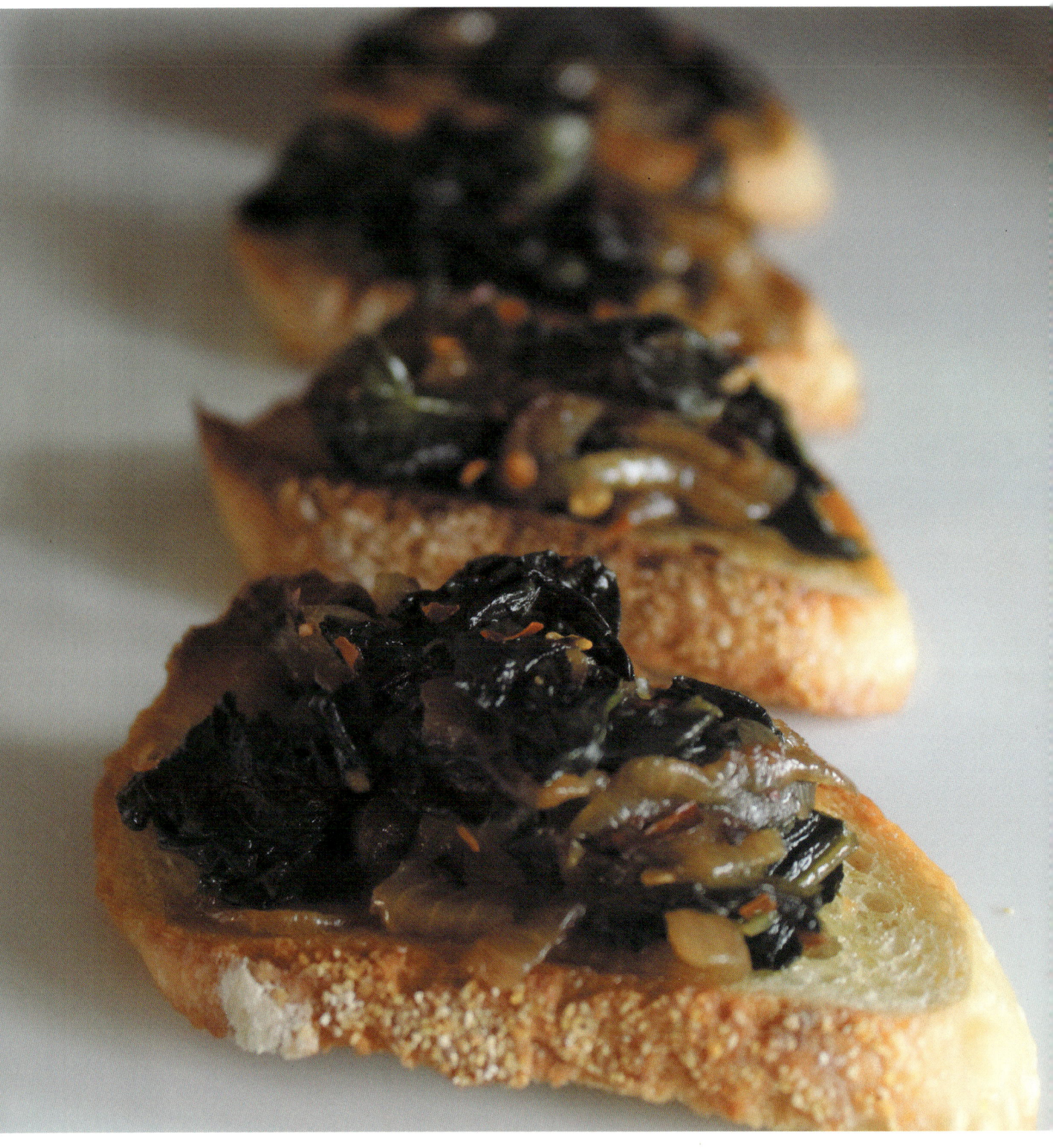

BLACK KALE CROSTINI WITH GARLIC, LEMON AND RED PEPPER FLAKES

Crostini di Cavolo Nero con Aglio, Limone e Peperoncino

Serves 4–5

Cavolo Nero is one of our favorite vegetables—not just because of the overall taste, but also for its nutritional value and versatility; we can adapt it to many different recipes, as we have done in this book. It is also very easy to grow; we always have it in our garden at home.

Cavolo Nero is part of the cabbage family but does not form a central head as the regular green cabbage does. Black or Tuscan kale is sweeter than the other varieties such as the Curly Kale that is commonly found in stores; other varieties include the Purple and Red Russian Kales.

This is a simple yet flavorful appetizer.

Ingredients

2 bunches black kale, trimmed and shredded (approximately 6 cups)

Approximately 3 tablespoons of extra virgin olive oil

3–4 large garlic cloves, sliced

Dry red pepper flakes to taste

Zest of 2 large lemons

Sea salt

1 baguette, sliced

Pre-heat the oven to 375°F.

Wash the kale and trim away the tough center stalk, then shred remaining kale leaves.

In a large pan, heat up three tablespoons of olive oil over medium heat. Add the garlic and red pepper flakes; cook only until the garlic releases its aroma, then add the kale and lemon zest. Thoroughly combine, season with salt, and continue mixing until the kale has completely wilted and released it juices. Set aside without draining.

Slice the baguette into half-inch slices and rub them with some olive oil. Place the bread on a large cookie sheet and toast them in the oven for about 10–15 minutes or until golden brown; keep an eye on the bread as they could burn easily, especially if cut too thin. Remove from the oven and let them cool completely before assembling.

Top each slice with the kale, letting the bread absorb some of the moisture. Drizzle with olive oil and serve.

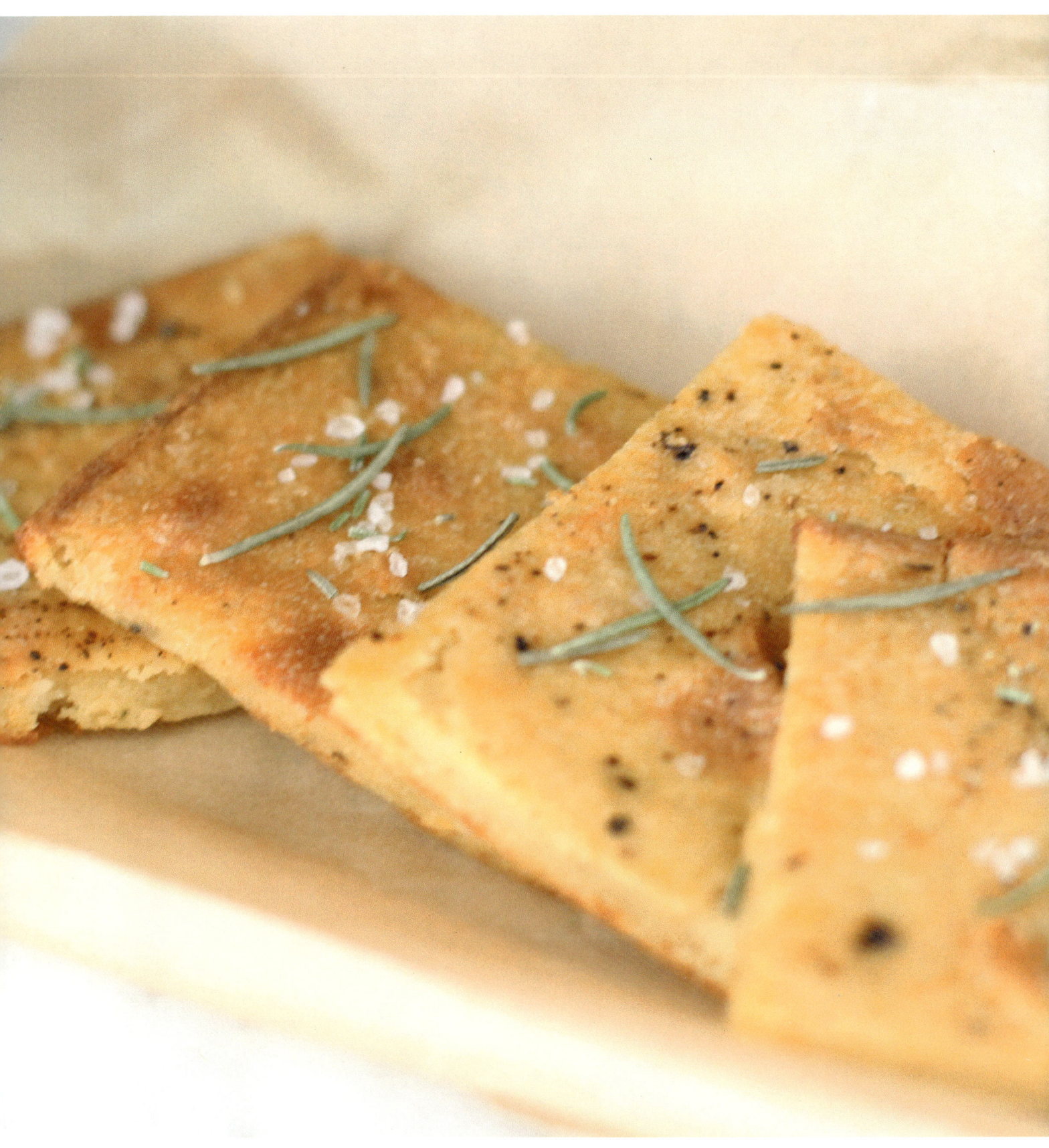

CHICKPEA FLATBREAD

Cecina, Torta di Ceci

Makes 1–2 flatbreads

Cecina is a traditional food from Pisa and Livorno. It's also known as *torta di ceci* or *farinata*, and is called *faina* in the coastal province of Savona; in Nice, France, it is called *socca*. Made with chickpea flour, olive oil, and water, cecina is best eaten right after it comes out of the oven. It is often sold at pizzerias stuffed in a piece of focaccia bread. In Liguria, they add rosemary or onions to the batter, and sometimes cheese or cured meats so that it becomes a fuller meal.

It's best to let the batter rest for at least four hours or overnight; it helps minimize the acidity of the flour.

Ingredients

2 cups chickpea or garbanzo flour

2¼ cups water

1 teaspoon of sea salt, or more if needed

½ cup extra virgin olive oil

1½ teaspoon of freshly ground black pepper

1 tablespoon of fresh rosemary, chopped (optional)

In a large bowl, mix the flour with a wooden spoon. Slowly add the water while stirring, making sure to eliminate any lumps. Add the salt and olive oil. The mixture should be very smooth and liquid.

Cover and let the mixture rest for at least four hours or overnight. Remove any foam that has formed at the top and mix again.

Heat oven to 400°F. Using a large baking pan with low borders, pour some olive oil into baking pan and add the mixture, making sure it is fairly low in the pan. The cecina has to be no thicker than half an inch high; if your pan is not large enough, you may need to bake two separate batches.

Bake for 35–40 minutes and remove from oven. Serve while warm.

SIDE DISHES

Contorni

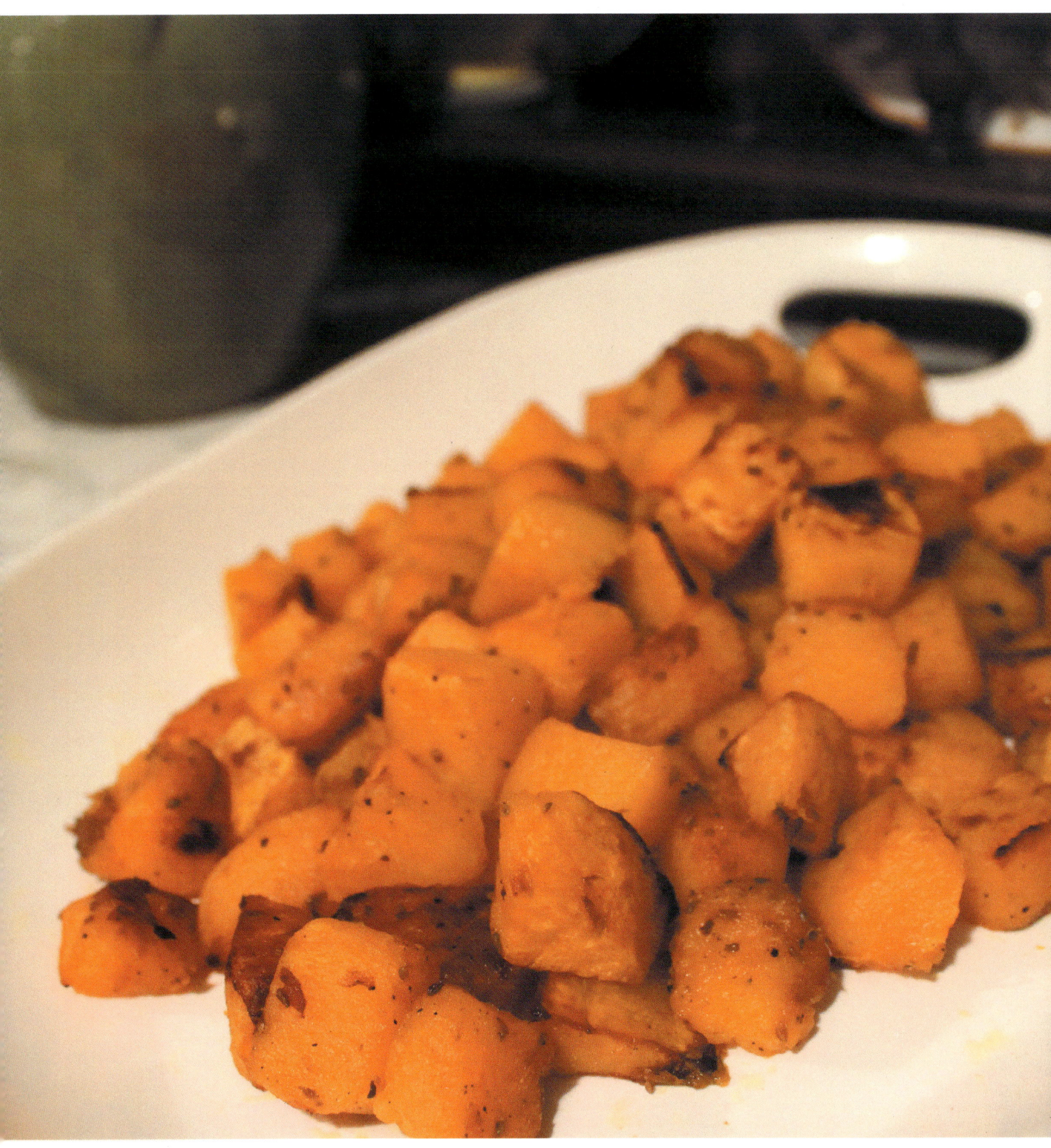

ROASTED BUTTERNUT SQUASH WITH OLIVE OIL AND ANISE

Zucca al Forno con Anice

Serves 4

Soon after the harvest, squashes were delivered to the big house by the dozens; some were cooked cut in large slices in a brown sugar syrup with allspice, and others were put into soups and pastas. The seeds were dried under the sun, and were later ground and turned into a delicious ancient sauce.

This recipe merges anise with brown sugar and olive oil, creating a hearty fall dish that goes well with roasted meats. Anise is commonly used in baked goods throughout Italy, from anicini and pizzelli cookies to liqueurs like Anesone and Sambuca.

Ingredients

1 large butternut squash, 3 pounds, cut into 2-inch cubes

1 tablespoon of anise seeds

4 tablespoons of extra virgin olive oil

3 tablespoons of brown sugar

A pinch of sea salt

A pinch of freshly ground black pepper

Pre-heat the oven to 385°F, placing oven rack on second-top position.

In a large mixing bowl, combine all the ingredients until the butternut cubes are evenly covered. Place the squash in a large baking pan, in a single layer, and roast for about 30–35 minutes. During the roasting time, shake the pan and rotate the pieces of squash with a large wooden spoon. When the butternut squash is slightly soft and a little brown on the edges, remove from the oven and serve hot.

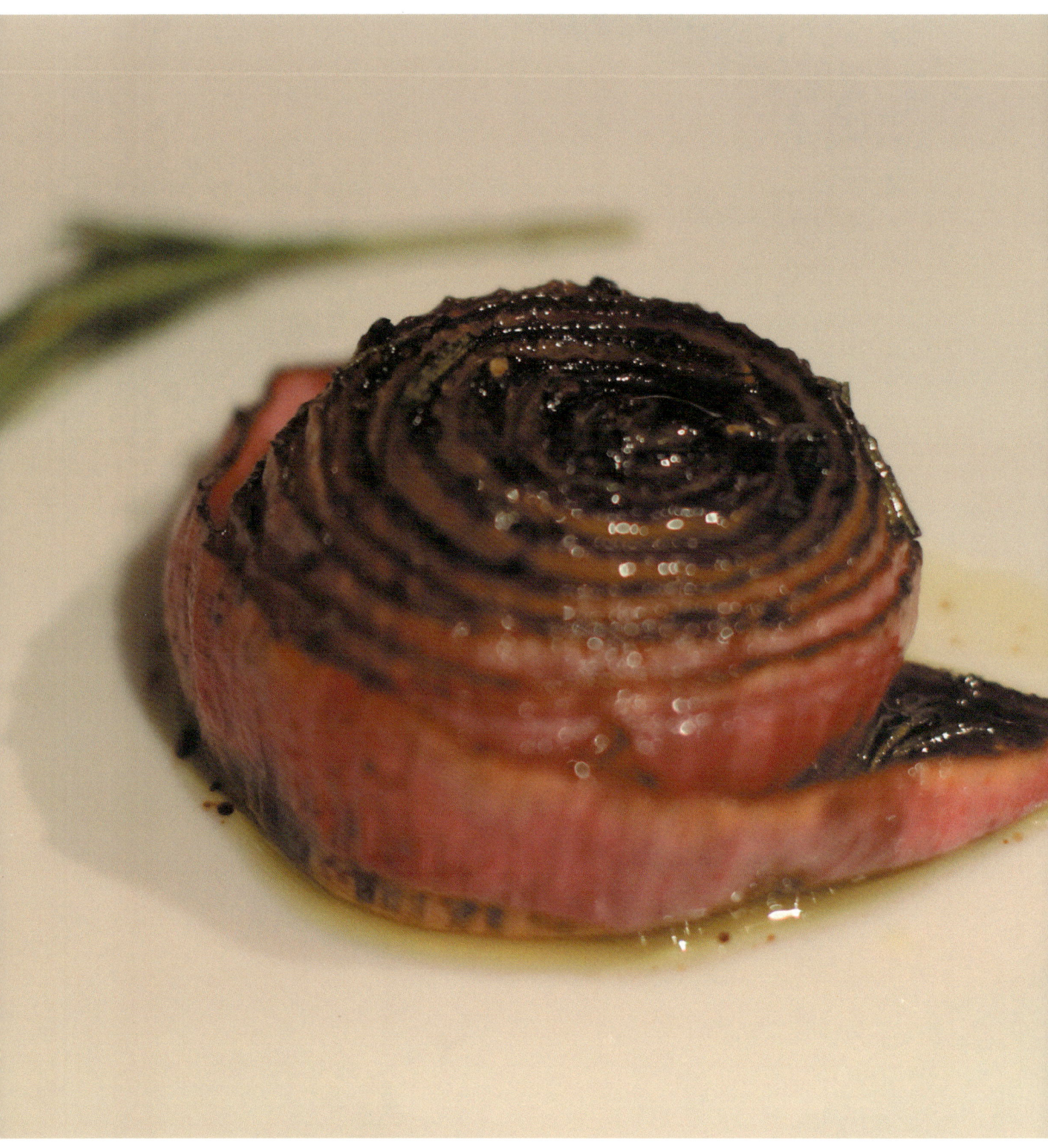

ROASTED RED ONIONS WITH BALSAMIC AND ROSEMARY

Cipolle all'Aceto Balsamico e Rosmarino

Serves 4

Red onions are simply exquisite when accompanied with balsamic vinegar and fresh rosemary. They go well with roasted meats, fish, or on a bed of mashed cannellini beans.

Ingredients

½ cup balsamic vinegar

½ cup extra virgin olive oil

Sea salt and black pepper to taste

4 medium-size red onions, cut in half, 2¼–2½ pounds

1 tablespoon fresh rosemary, finely chopped

Pre-heat oven to 425°F.

In a small bowl, mix the balsamic vinegar and olive oil. Season with salt and pepper, and set aside.

On a baking pan, arrange onions in one layer, cut side up, and drizzle the balsamic, olive oil mixture, and the rosemary over top; roast in the middle of the pre-heated oven until golden brown, about 20–25 minutes. At this point, the balsamic vinegar will reduce and onions will be tender. Add more balsamic mix during roasting if the onions appear to become to dry. Remove from the oven.

Serve at room temperature.

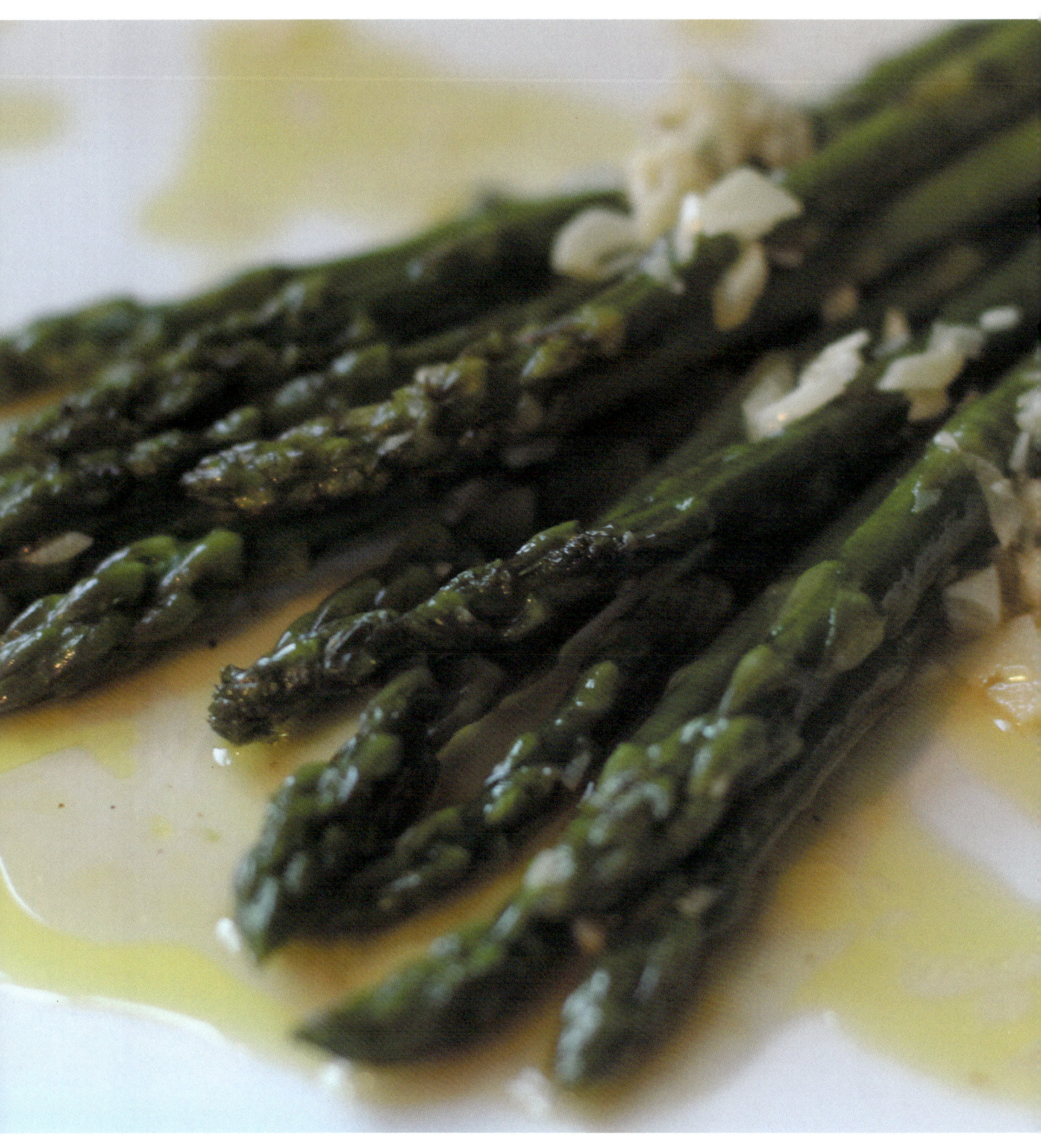

ASPARAGUS WITH GARLIC

Asparagi con Aglio

Serves 3–4

Here is a recipe for a simple side dish—asparagus sautéed in olive oil and lots of garlic.

Ingredients

2 tablespoons extra virgin olive oil

1 bunch fresh asparagus, washed, with white ends cut off

4 large cloves garlic, minced

Sea salt

Ground black pepper or red pepper flakes to taste

Heat the olive oil in a frying pan over medium-high heat; add the asparagus and cook for 8–10 minutes, stirring frequently. When asparagus is done, quickly add the garlic and season with salt, pepper, and/or red pepper flakes to taste. Do not let the garlic brown; it will be ready as soon it starts releasing its aroma.

Remove from heat and serve.

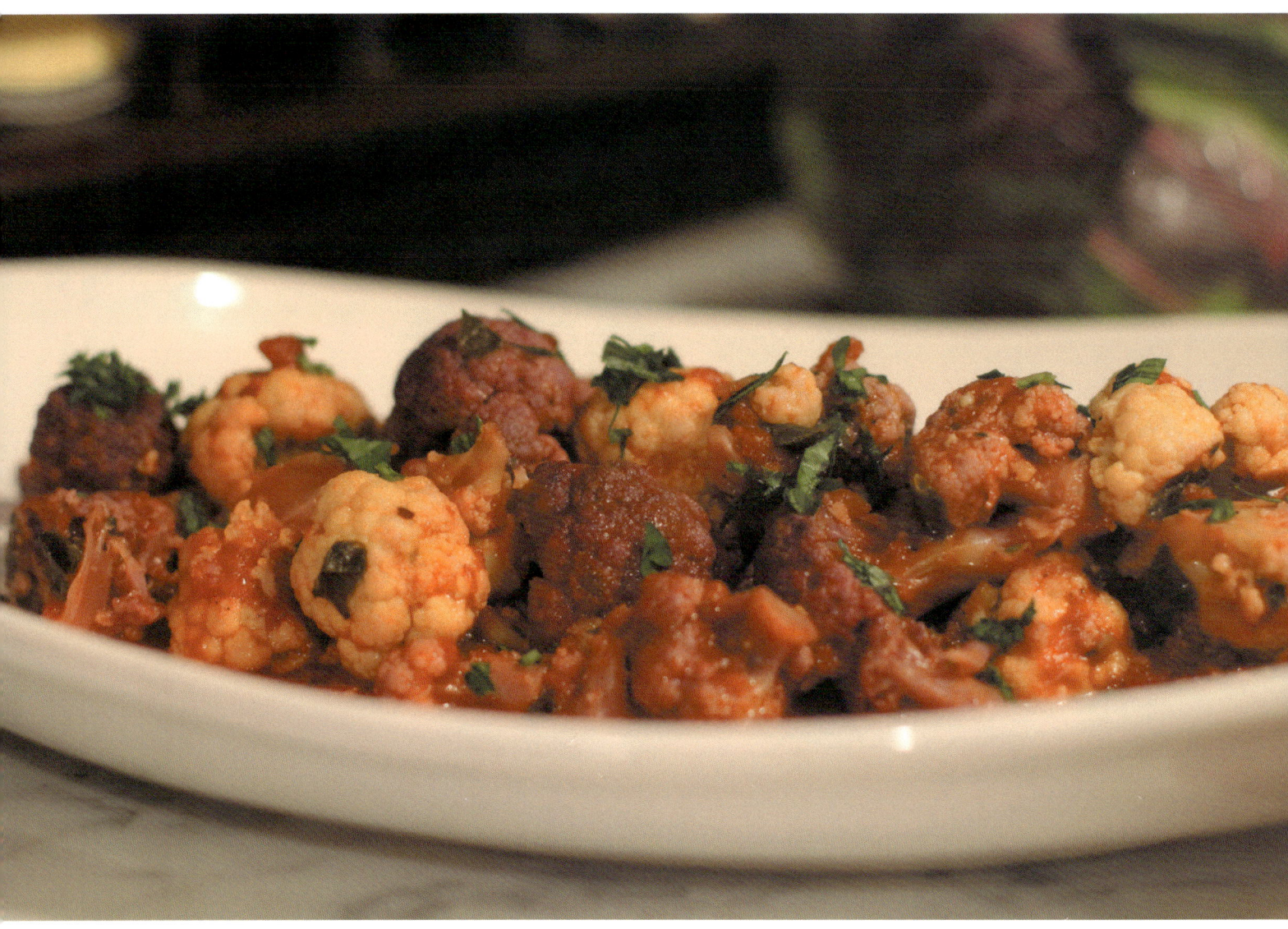

STEWED CAULIFLOWER
Cavolfiore Stufato

Serves 4

During the cabbage harvest in late October and November, cauliflower was so abundant in the house that it was served as an after-school snack, simply boiled and served with a sour cream sauce. It also showed up in many other manifestations, such as fritters, tortilla, salad, and soups; later, when we were in Italy, it was cooked into risotto.

Tuscans usually boil cauliflower before incorporating into other dishes or other condiments. This recipe keeps cooking to a minimum, just enough to leave the cauliflower with a crisp bite.

For this recipe we like to use purple, white, and yellow cauliflower; the purple variety of cauliflower comes from Italy or South Africa, and has a milder, sweeter, nuttier taste than white. Yellow cauliflower began as a result of a naturally occurring mutation that first showed up in Canada.

Ingredients

2 medium-size cauliflowers, colored or white

4 tablespoons of extra virgin olive oil

2 garlic cloves, finely chopped

Red pepper flakes or freshly ground black pepper

1½ cups Italian chopped tomatoes

Sea salt

1 cup of chopped fresh basil

Water, 1 cup, if needed

Parboil the cauliflower for five minutes in salted water, and then break it into bite-size florets. Cauliflower is usually parboiled to reduce the smell, which many find too strong.

In a large pan, heat the oil on medium-high heat, add the garlic and pepper flakes, and sauté very briefly, just enough to let the garlic release its aroma. Add the chopped tomatoes and basil and cook for about 10 minutes. Add some of the water to thin the sauce, season with salt, and add the cauliflower, turning it over gently.

Cook for five minutes so the flavors combine; taste for salt, and drizzle some extra virgin olive oil.

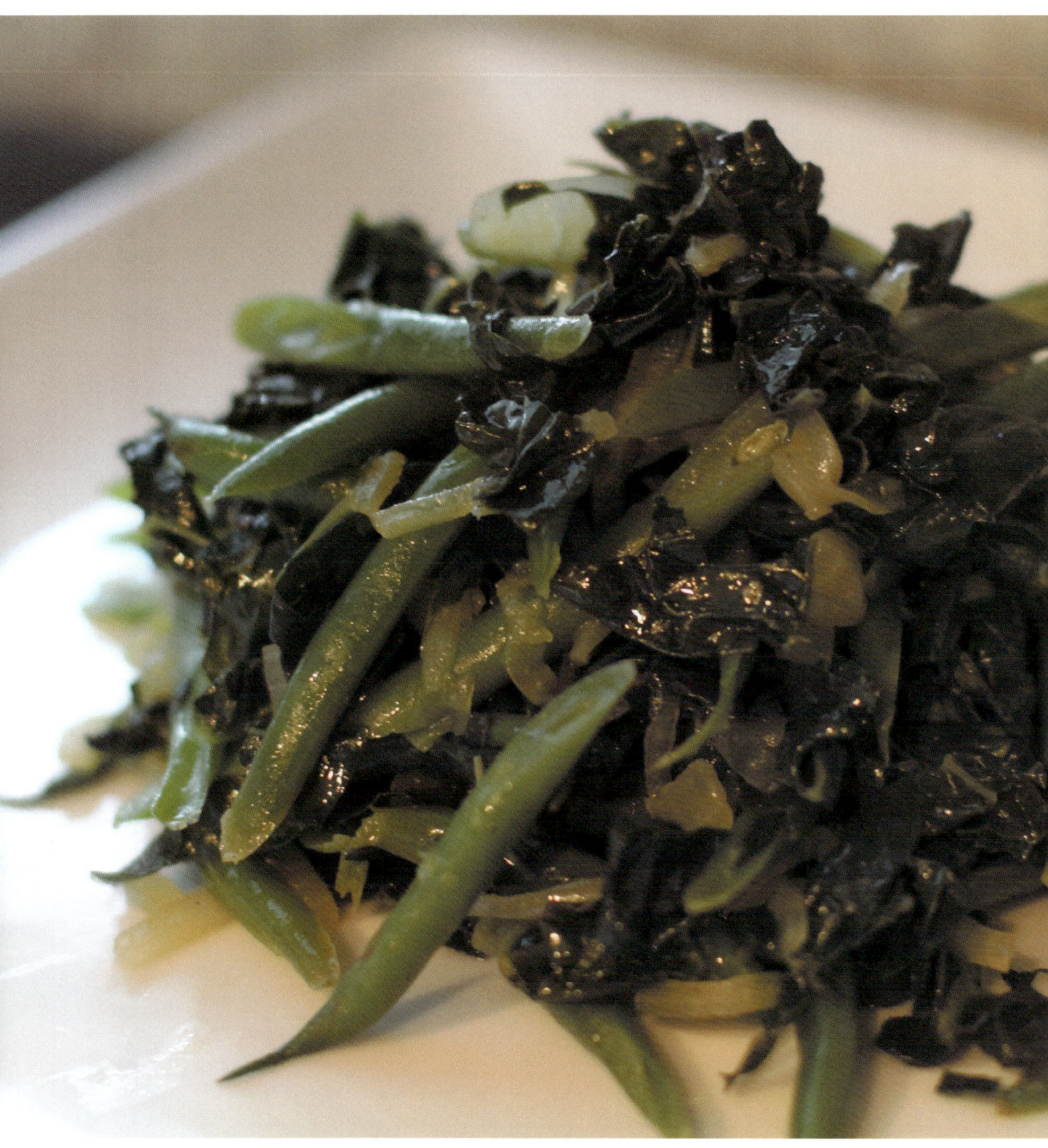

BLACK KALE WITH STRING BEANS AND FRESH BASIL

Cavolo Nero con Fagolini e Basilico

Serves 4-5

Until recently, Cavolo Nero, or Tuscan Kale, was one of Italy's best kept secrets. Simply adored, especially in the north of Italy, it has been an essential fare with, or as part of, traditional dishes for centuries. We never get tired of it, and make a dish with kale just about every week.

Cavolo Nero is an essential ingredient in the famous Tuscan soup, Ribollita, the "re-boiled" bean soup thickened with bread and drizzled with olive oil. It can be used, as with most Italian ingredients, in an extensive array of dishes, including risotto, pasta, and frittata. In this recipe, it is sautéed and combined with green beans in good olive oil, and flavored with garlic, basil, red pepper flakes and sea salt. As you can see from this recipe, it reflects the Italian method of using a few—but the best quality—ingredients.

Ingredients

1 pound of green beans, trimmed

Extra virgin olive oil

2 garlic cloves, finely chopped

Red pepper flakes

1 pound of kale, chopped

1 cup fresh basil, chopped

Sea salt

Bring a large pot full of salted water to a boil and cook the green beans for about five minutes. Remove beans from the water and place immediately in cold water to stop the cooking. Green beans should have a crunch, so do not overcook. Let them cool completely, then drain.

In a large pan, heat the olive oil under medium heat. Add the garlic until it releases its fragrance; add the red pepper flakes, kale, and basil; mix well and sauté until the kale is tender. Add the string beans to the kale and combine well, and season with salt.

Serve hot.

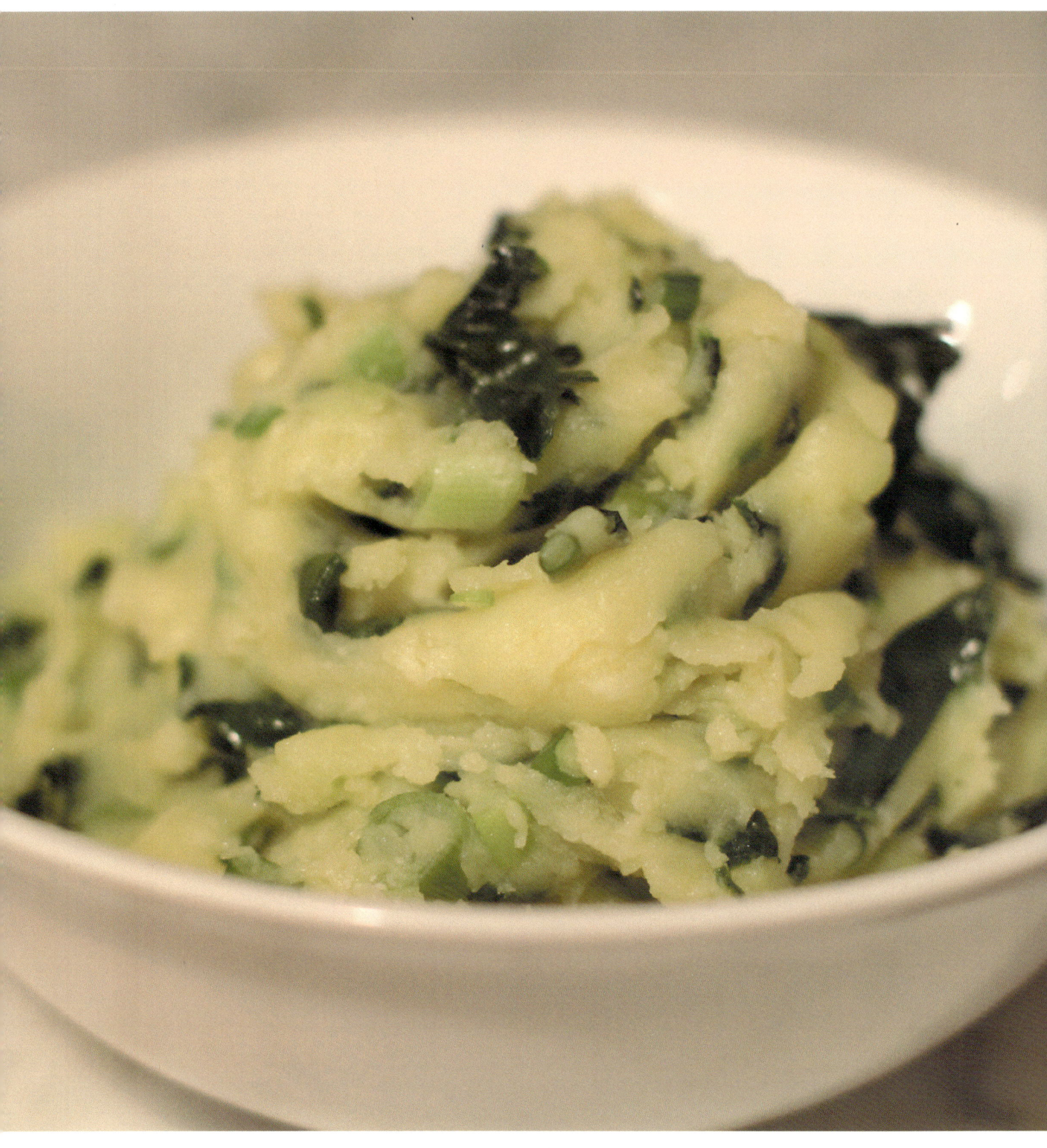

MASHED POTATOES WITH KALE, BASIL, AND GARLIC

Puré di Patate con Cavolo Nero

Serves 4-5

Potatoes took a long time to catch on. Though they were introduced to Italy in 1585 via Spain, they weren't taken seriously as a food crop until the 1800s as they were considered poisonous, evil, and the cause of many diseases. However, they have made up for lost time, and are now a staple on the Italian table.

These potatoes are the perfect comfort side dish to any steak or chicken.

Ingredients

3 pounds potatoes, such as Yukon gold

⅓ cup extra virgin olive oil (plus 1 tablespoon to sauté the garlic and kale)

3 garlic cloves, minced

1 bunch black kale

1 cup buttermilk or whole milk, at room temperature

½ cup grated Parmesan

Sea salt

Freshly ground pepper

Put the potatoes into a large pot and cover them completely with water. Add a few pinches of salt and bring the water to a boil. Cook until the potatoes are tender, 20–25 minutes. Drain, cool, and peel.

While the potatoes cook, heat the one tablespoon of olive oil and the garlic in a small sauté pan over medium-low heat; sauté the garlic until it releases its aroma. Add the kale and combine. Season with salt and cook until wilted, then set aside.

Put the potatoes in a large mixing bowl; using a potato masher, mash the potatoes together with the ⅓ cup olive oil and milk (or buttermilk) until you get a smooth consistency. Add the sautéed kale to the potatoes, and season with salt and pepper to taste. Adjust the amount of milk (or buttermilk) to your preferred consistency.

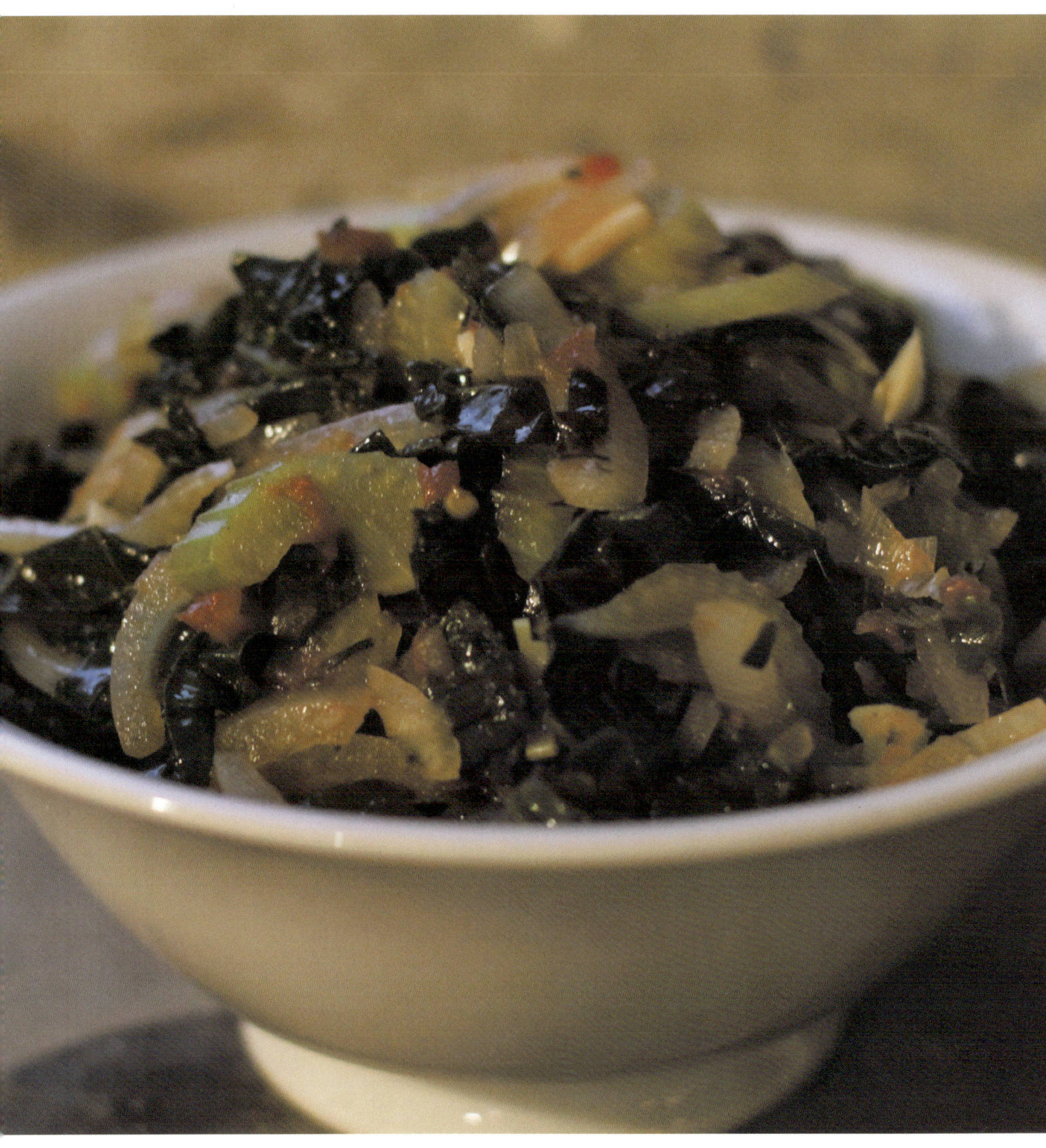

KALE WITH LEEKS, CELERY, AND TOMATOES

Kale con Porri, Sedano, e Pomodori

Serves 4–5

We love black kale so much that even our dogs, Bailey and Griffin, have developed a taste for fresh herbs and vegetables—from fresh basil, kale, celery, avocados, fresh fruits, and fresh corn, among others.

This is a quick, hearty, and satisfying recipe—and extremely healthy as well.

Ingredients

4 tablespoons of olive oil

2 cloves of garlic, finely chopped

Red pepper flakes

1 cup chopped Italian tomatoes

Sea salt

4–6 celery stalks cut into thin slices

2 leeks, rinsed and cut into thin half-moons

4 cups of black kale, chopped, trimmed, veins removed

In a large sauté pan, heat 2 tablespoons olive oil at medium-high heat. Add the garlic and pepper flakes to taste, just until the garlic releases its aroma; do not brown. Add the tomatoes, season with salt, and cook just for five minutes.

Remove from the pan and set aside.

Using the same pan, return to medium-high heat and add the remaining 2 tablespoons of olive oil; add the celery and leeks. Cook just long enough for them remain crisp. Add the kale and continue cooking until wilted, then add the sauce and combine well.

Adjust the salt and pepper flakes to taste.

Remove from pan and drizzle with some additional olive oil.

Serve warm.

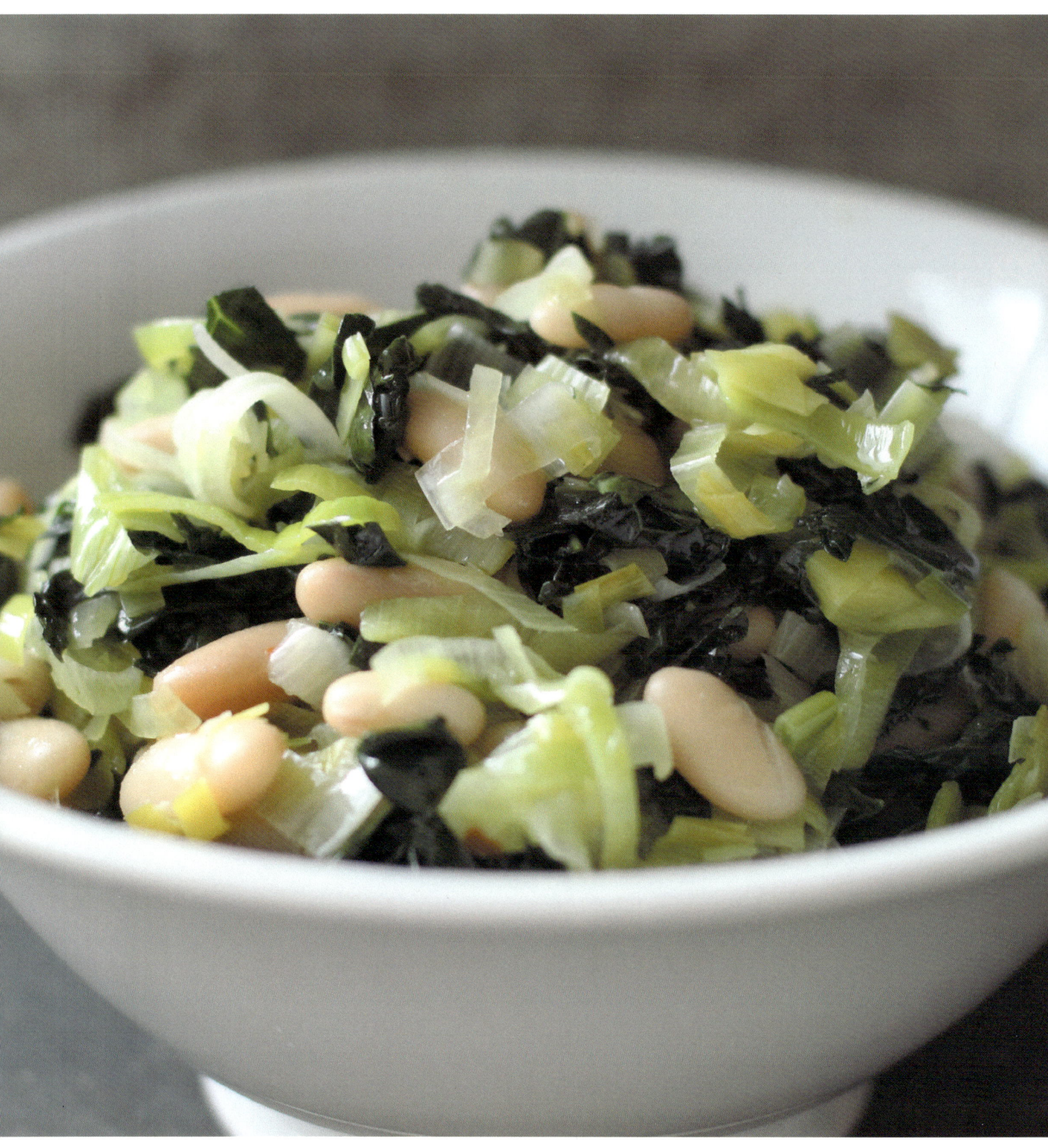

BLACK KALE WITH LEEKS AND CANNELLINI BEANS

Cavolo Nero con Porri e Fagioli

Serves 4–5

Kale and creamy cannellini beans make a wonderful side dish and serve as a hearty vegetarian entrée or side dish for any meal.

Ingredients

1 bunch black kale, ribs removed, leaves thinly sliced crosswise

4 tablespoons extra virgin olive oil

3 garlic cloves, thinly sliced

Sea salt

Ground pepper to taste

2–3 leeks cut in half-moons

1 (19 ounces) can of cannellini beans, drained and rinsed

½ cup of chicken or vegetable broth

Wash the kale and trim away the tough center stalk, then shred remaining kale leaves.

In a large pan, heat up three tablespoons of olive oil at medium heat; add the garlic and cook only until the garlic releases its aroma. Then add the kale, thoroughly combine, season with salt and pepper, and continue mixing until the kale has completely wilted and released it juices. Set aside without draining.

Using the same pan, warm one tablespoon of olive oil over medium heat; add the leeks and cook, stirring occasionally, until softened and translucent, about 10 minutes. Add the beans and a half-cup of broth, and season with salt and pepper to taste.

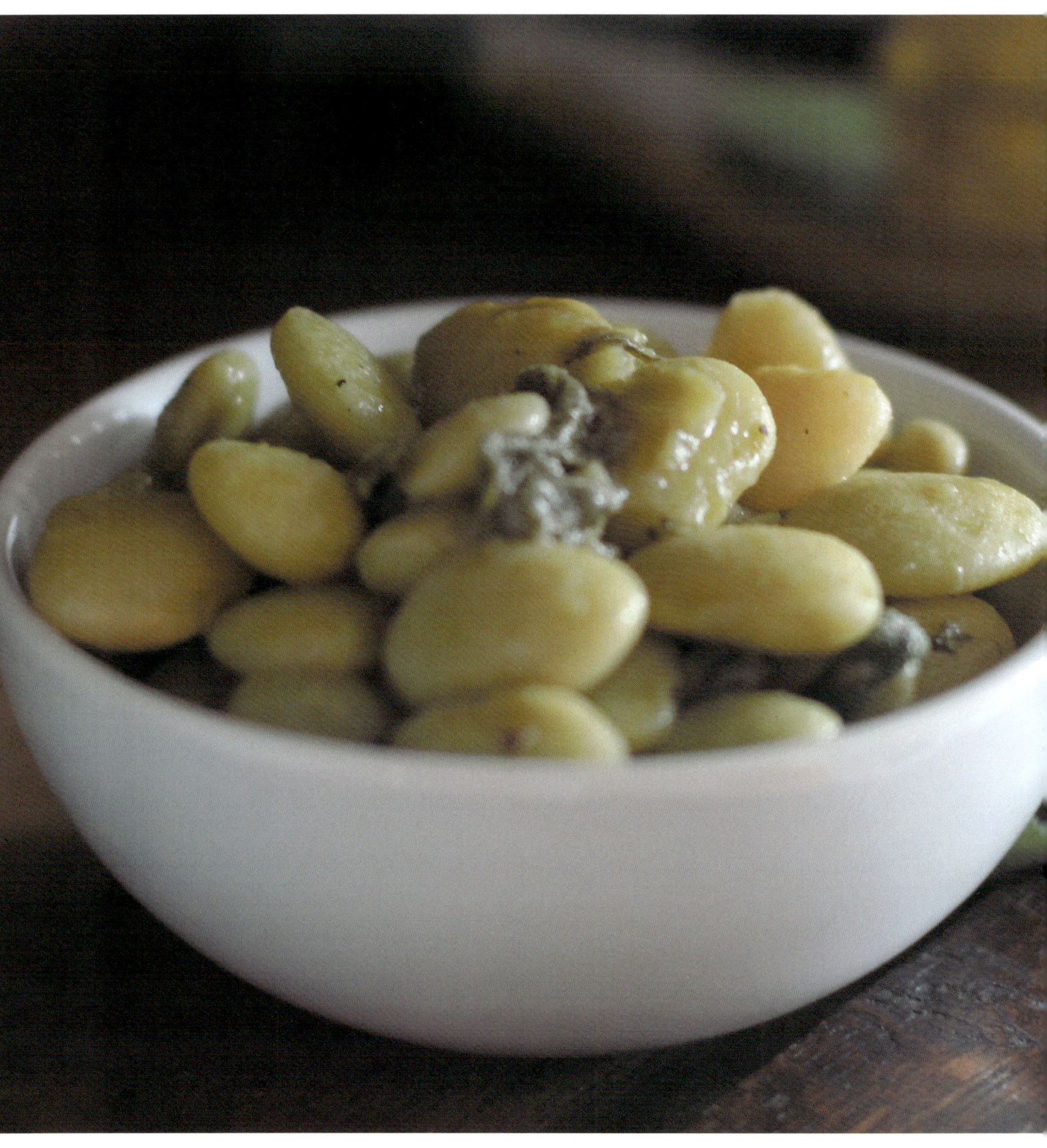

LIMA BEANS WITH SAGE

Fagiolo di Spagna Bollite con Salvia

Serves 4

This simple side dish will be a colorful addition to any menu. The combination of two flavors, fresh sage and extra virgin olive oil, enhances the beans, creating a delightful taste. The lima beans should still have a little bite, but are still tender and creamy.

Ingredients

1 pound frozen baby lima beans

1 cup water

4 tablespoons extra virgin olive oil

6–8 fresh sage leaves

Sea salt

Freshly ground black pepper

Rinse the frozen lima beans under cold running water and place in a pot. Add the water, which should be enough to cover the beans. Add three tablespoons of olive oil and the sage leaves, and season with salt and pepper.

Bring to a simmer and cook for about 15 minutes, stirring gently. When the beans are tender, remove from heat and drizzle with the remaining olive oil. Adjust salt and pepper to taste.

Serve warm or cold.

The Spanish brought "new" world dry beans—along with corn, tomatoes, pepper, potatoes, chocolate and cotton—back to the "old" world. Beans became a central part of the cuisine in Italy, Spain, and France. Beans are so important to Tuscan cuisine that they refer to themselves as the *mangiafagioli*—"the bean eaters." Florence, in fact, was the first Italian city to consider the New World fruits and vegetables as edibles while the rest of Italy saw them as ornamentals.

The region of Tuscany is famous for its bean production; cannellini and white kidney beans are perhaps the most popular; these are simply referred to as *fagioli*.

Here is both the quick method (using canned beans) and the traditional method of soaking the beans overnight. Both are simple, yet satisfying and full of flavor.

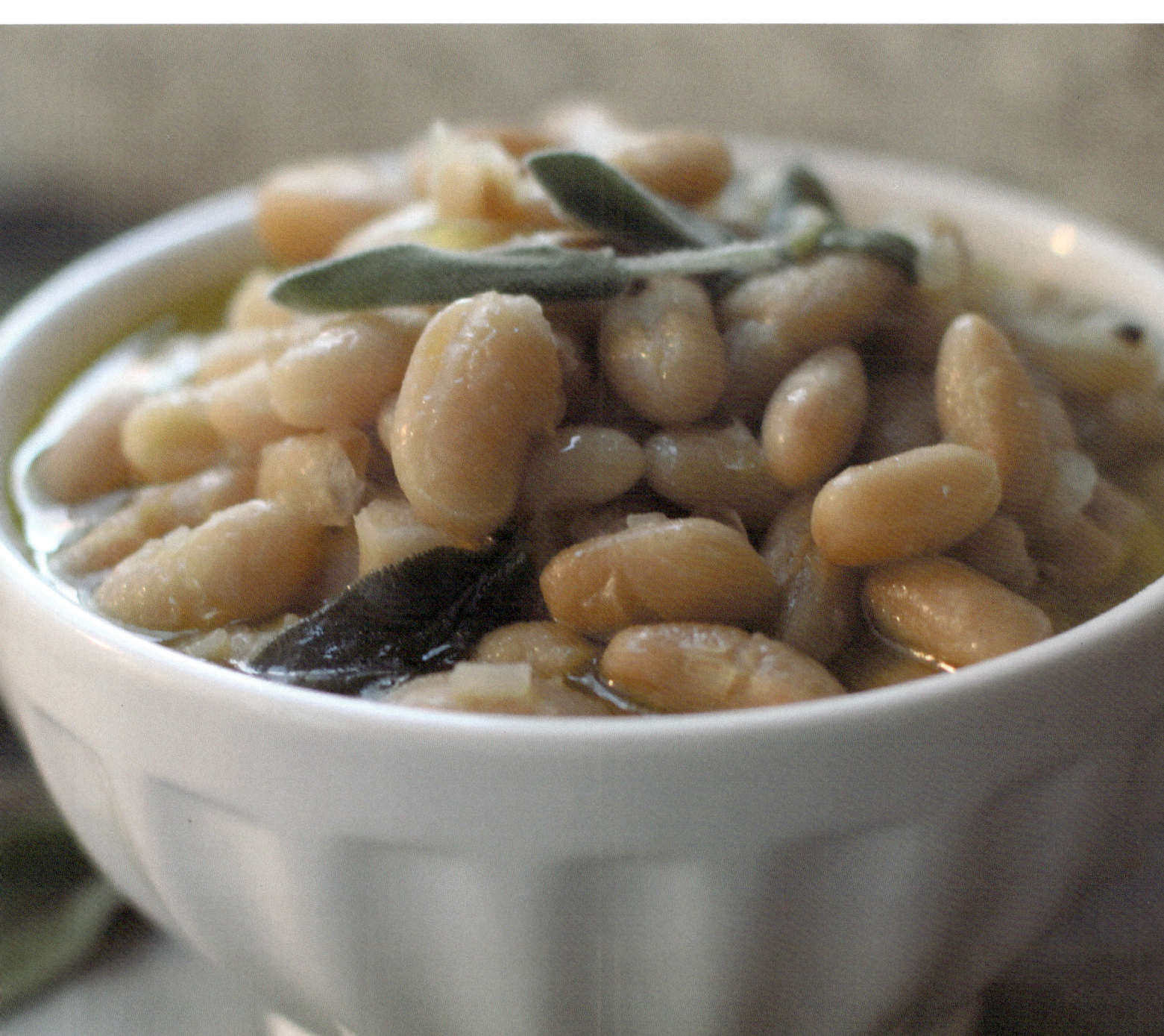

CANELLINI BEANS WITH FRESH SAGE, TUSCAN STYLE

Fagioli alla Toscana

Serves 4–5

Quick method:	**Traditional method:**
Ingredients	Ingredients
4 tablespoons extra virgin olive oil	1 pound dried cannellini beans
4 large garlic cloves, minced	12 cups cold water
3 tablespoons fresh sage, chopped	6 tablespoons extra virgin olive oil
2 (14 ounces) cans cannellini beans, drained and rinsed	1 teaspoon black pepper
Sea salt and pepper	4 large cloves garlic, lightly crushed
1 cup water or chicken stock	5–6 fresh sage leaves
	Sea salt and freshly ground black pepper.

In a large skillet, heat the olive oil at medium heat; add the garlic and sage and sauté just enough to release the garlic aroma. Add the beans and water (or chicken stock), season with salt and pepper, and cook until the beans are completely heated through. Remove from heat and serve.

This is the most popular way to prepare beans in Tuscany.

Clean the beans from any debris or stones then rinse them under cold running water. Put beans in a large pot, cover with cold water, and set aside to soak for at least five to six hours or overnight. Older beans take longer to soften.

Drain beans, then add 12 cups of cold water, three tablespoons of the oil, and the pepper, garlic, and sage. Cover the pot and bring to a simmer over medium heat for about one hour. Season with salt, reduce heat to medium-low, and gently simmer for one or two hours longer, stirring occasionally, until bean are tender.

Remove from heat, set aside, and allow beans to cool in the cooking liquid. To serve, reheat beans in their liquid and drizzle with the remaining three tablespoons of olive oil.

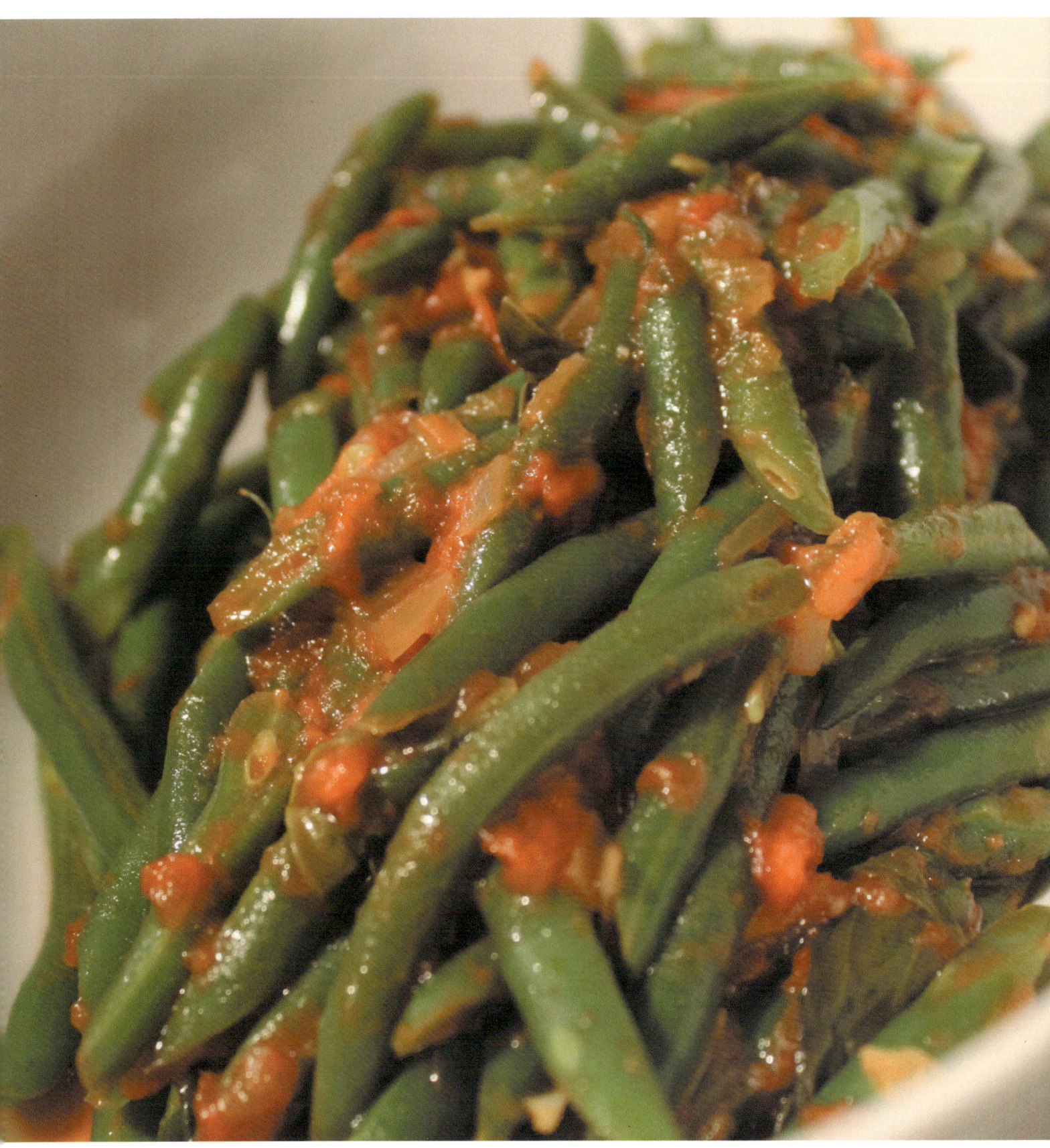

STEWED STRING BEANS IN TOMATO SAUCE

Umido di Fagiolini in Salsa di Pomodoro

Serves 4–5

I remember this recipe very well from my youth. I associate string beans with the women of the house congregating over a large basket full of them, brought by relatives from the north. With much laughter, they discussed politics, sorrows and pains, and the latest gossip while preparing the beans for a variety of dishes. The beans were turned into soups, stews, sautés, and omelets, among other dishes.

Ingredients

1 pound fresh string beans, trimmed and cut

1 tablespoon extra virgin olive oil

1½ cups Quick Tomato Sauce with Fresh Basil (see recipe on page 7)

Sea salt

Prepare green beans and bring a pot of water to a boil. Allow green beans to boil for 4–5 minutes, ensuring they don't change color and lose their crispness.

Drain green beans and add to an ice water bath. Drain again and set aside until ready to sauté.

Heat the olive oil in a saucepan or skillet over medium heat. Add the green beans and tomato sauce; cook for 3–5 minutes. Season with salt and pepper to taste.

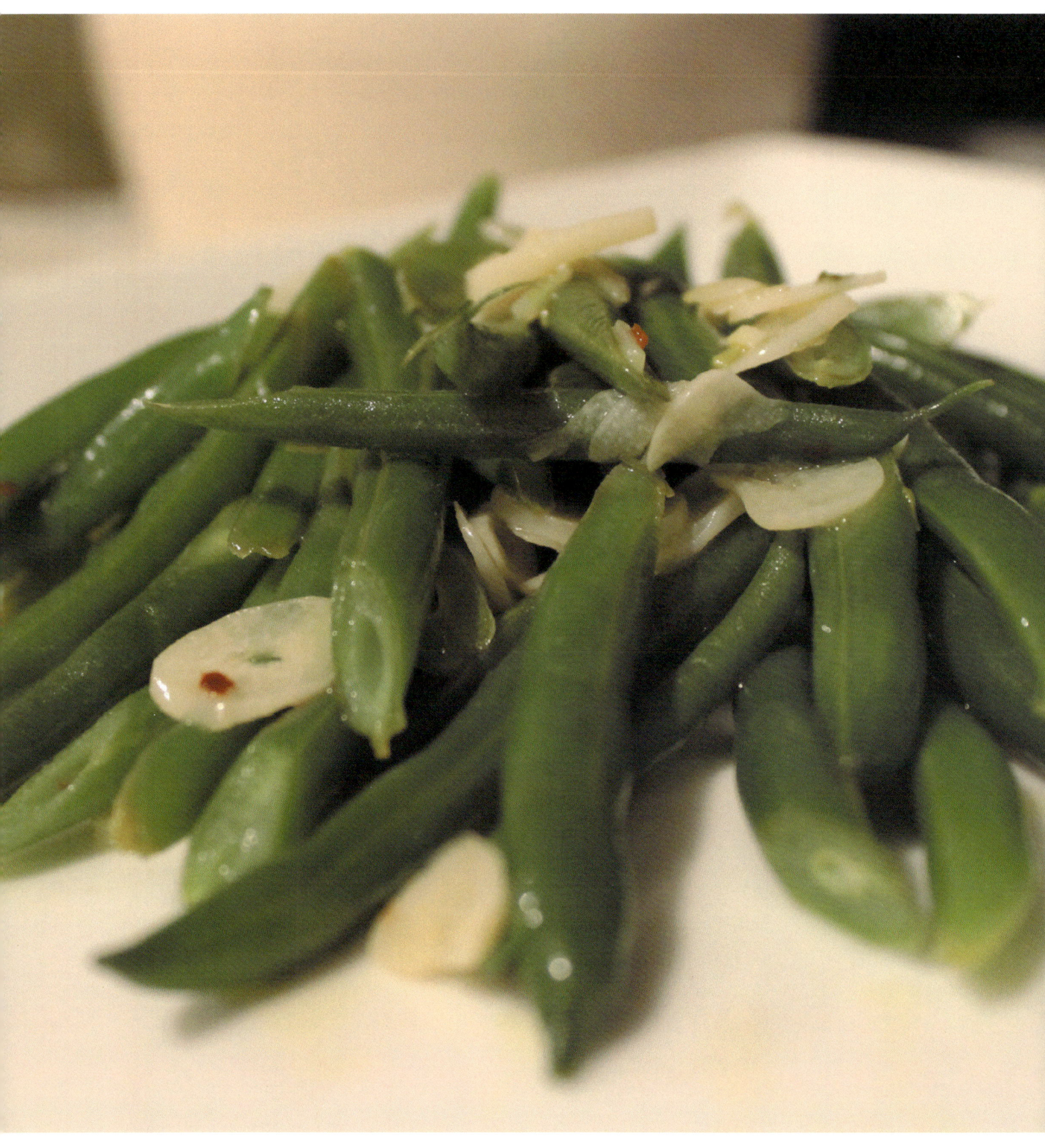

GARLICKY STRING BEANS
Fagiolini con Aglio

Serves 4–5

No ingredient seems more familiar with Italian cooking than garlic, but in reality, Italians don't use as much garlic as one may think. Nonna Maria used to serve this side dish loaded with barely cooked garlic, which imparted a mild flavor without being overpowering. The trick to obtaining a subtle garlic taste is to cook the garlic without browning it. This dish is similar to the Spanish tapas *judias verdes al ajillo*.

Ingredients

5–6 cups of water

Sea salt

1 to 1½ pounds of fresh string beans, trimmed

4 tablespoons of extra virgin olive oil
    plus 1–2 for drizzling

5 cloves of garlic, peeled and thinly sliced

Red pepper flakes

½ cup white wine

In a large pot, bring five to six cups of water to a boil. Add about a teaspoon of salt, then add the string beans; cook for five minutes. Remove from heat, drain, and dip into ice water to stop the cooking. Drain again when cool, then set aside.

In a large sauté pan, heat 4 tablespoons of olive oil to medium-high heat. Add the red pepper flakes to taste, then add the garlic; cook just for one minute. Add the wine and string beans, and cook just long enough for the alcohol to evaporate. Season with salt to taste.

Remove from heat, then drizzle with some more olive oil and serve hot.

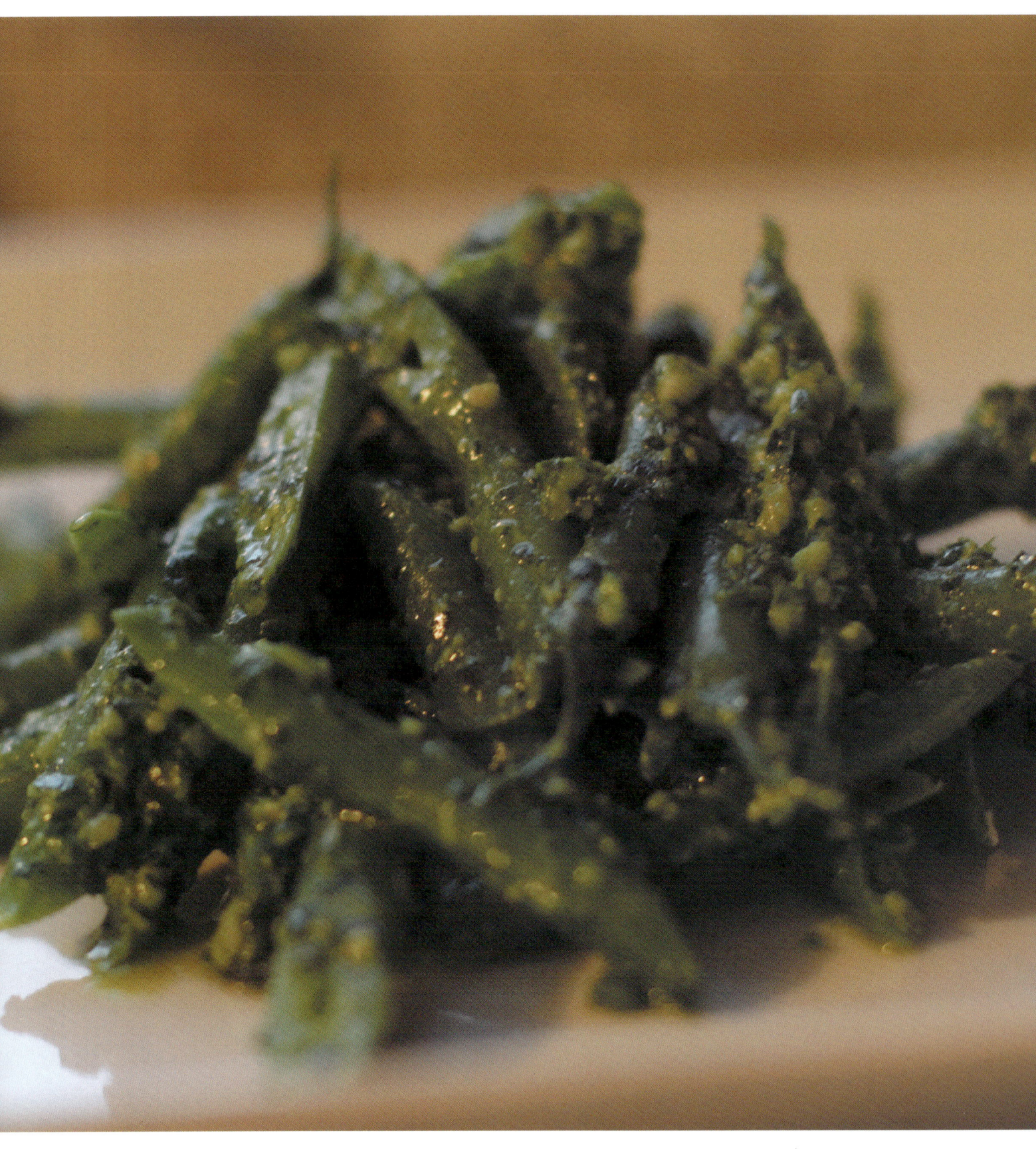

STRING BEANS WITH PARSLEY PESTO
Fagiolini con Pesto di Prezzemolo

Serves 4–5

String beans (*fagiolini*)—like peppers, tomatoes, and corn—are a gift of the Americas
to the old world. This recipe marries both
worlds, the ancient pesto with the string
beans, resulting in a delicious side dish.

Ingredients

1 pound fresh string beans, trimmed and cut

1½ cups Parsley Pesto
   (see recipe on page 5)

Prepare green beans and bring a pot of water to a boil. Allow green beans to boil for
four to five minutes, ensuring they don't change color and lose their crispness.

Drain green beans and add to an ice water bath. Drain and set aside until ready
to sauté.

Heat the Parsley Pesto in a saucepan or skillet on medium heat and add the green
beans. Cook for three to five minutes, until all the string beans are coated and
heated through.

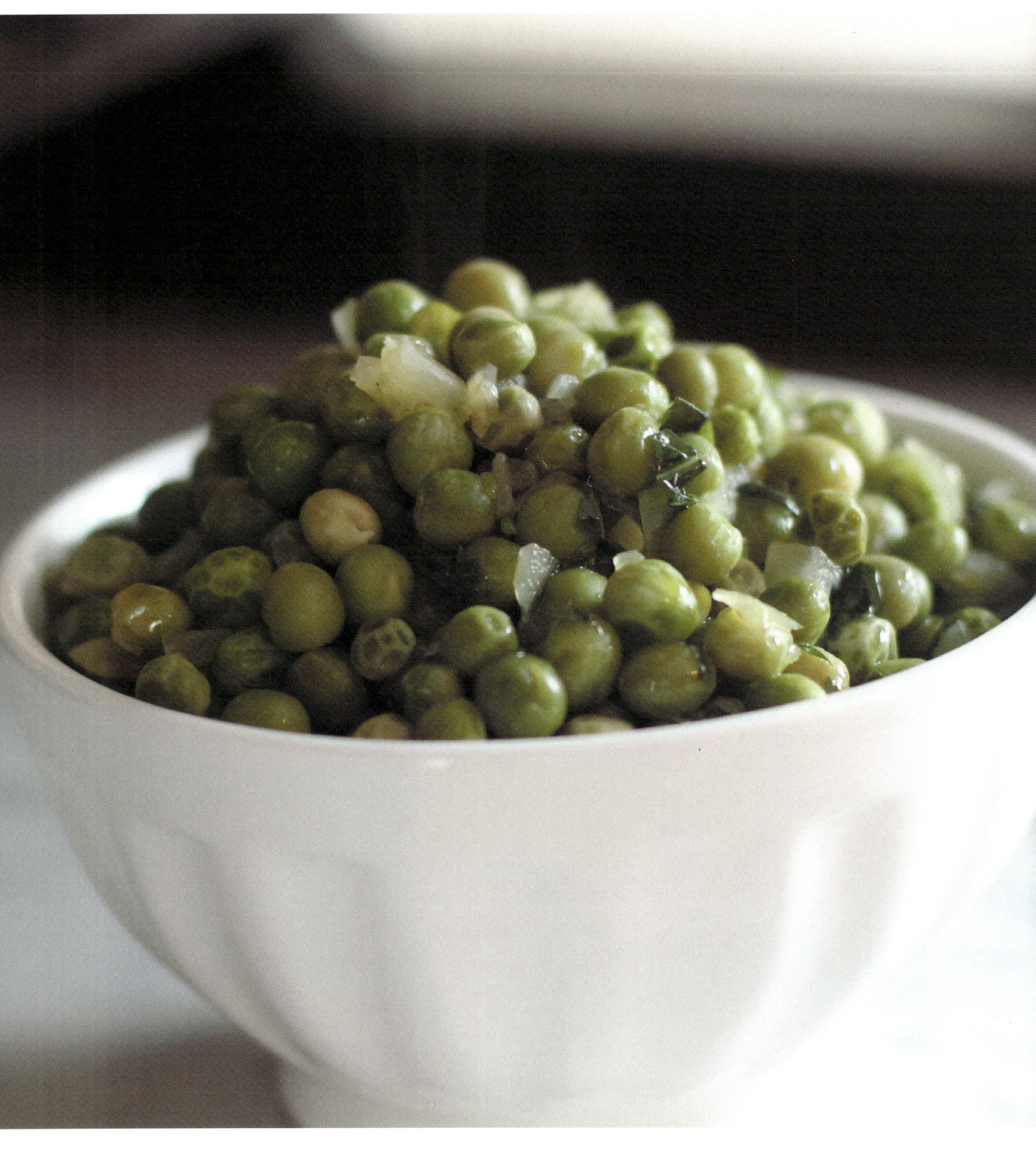

PEAS WITH ONIONS AND FRESH MINT

Piselli alla Menta

Serves 4

Piselli alla Fiorentina or Florentine style peas stewed with tomatoes is perhaps one of the most frequently served vegetable dishes in Florence—and also in our own home. In Tuscany the availability of fresh peas at the public markets is very short due to the short growing season. Here in the United States we use store-bought frozen peas and fresh mint available all year long to create a bright and healthy dish.

Ingredients

3 tablespoons of extra virgin olive oil

1 small onion, finely chopped

3 cups frozen peas

½ cup chopped fresh mint

1–2 cups water

Sea salt

Freshly ground black pepper

In a medium-size pot, heat the olive oil at medium heat, and sauté the onion until soft or translucent. Add the peas, mint, and one cup of water; season with salt and pepper to taste and bring to a simmer. Cook for 10–15 minutes, adjusting the amount of water if too dry.

Remove from heat and serve warm.

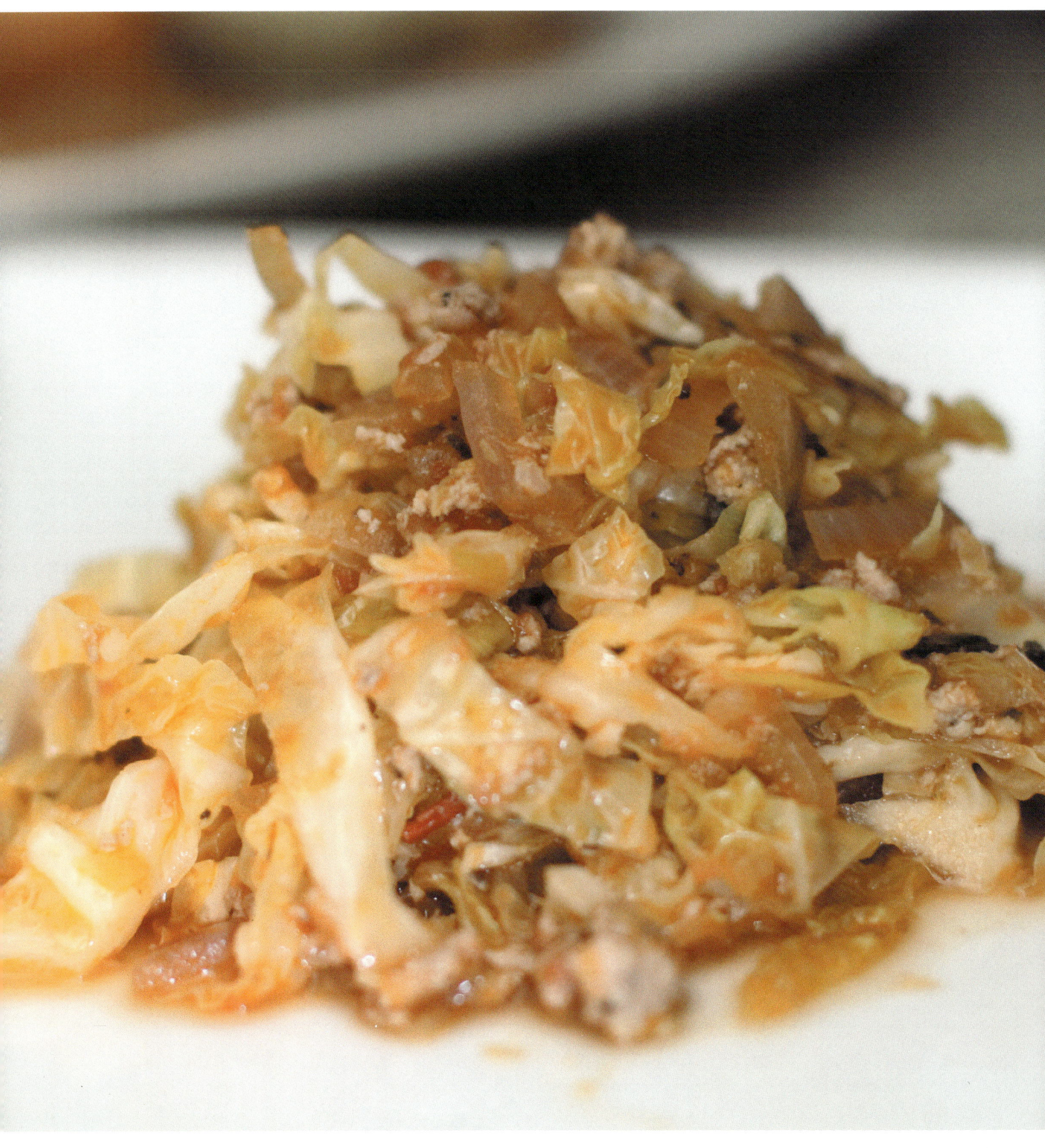

SAVOY CABBAGE WITH FRESH SAUSAGE

Cavolo Verza con Pomodori, e Salsicce Fresche

Serves 4–5

There are many delicious cabbage dishes across Italy such as this robust selection. Savoy cabbage, sausages, and tomatoes go extremely well together. This is basically a one-pot dish that develops a better flavor the following day.

Ingredients

1 pound Savoy cabbage, cored and shredded

3 tablespoons olive oil

1 pound of sausage meat, with or without fennel

1 large yellow onion, halved and cut into very thin rings

2 large garlic cloves, minced

1 cup chopped canned Italian plum tomatoes

½ cup chicken stock

Sea salt

Black pepper

Red pepper flakes to taste.

Remove the core of the cabbage and cut the remaining cabbage into quarter-inch strips. You should have about four firmly packed cups of cabbage strips.

Place the olive oil in a large sauté pan over medium heat. Add the sausage and cook until it starts to brown; add the onion rings, and sauté until they start to become translucent. Add the cabbage and garlic, stirring to blend well.

Add the tomatoes to the cabbage, chicken stock and season with sea salt and ground black pepper, as well as red pepper flakes to taste.

Bring mixture to a simmer, reduce heat, and cook, uncovered, for 20–25 minutes, or until cabbage is softened and flavors are blended.

When ready to serve, drizzle some extra virgin olive oil over the cabbage.

SALADS

Insalate

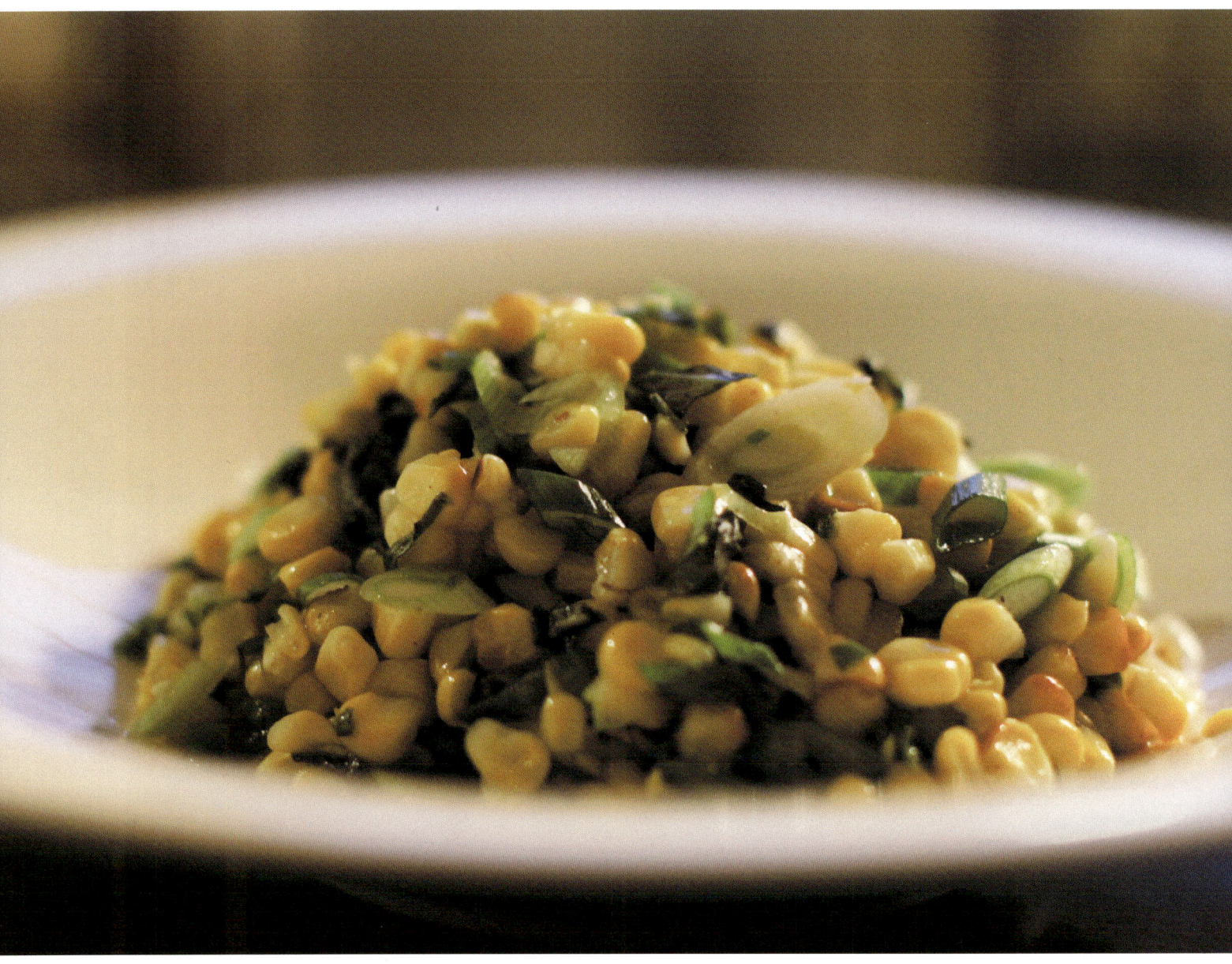

ROASTED CORN SALAD WITH SCALLIONS, BASIL, AND CUMIN LEMON DRESSING

Insalata di Mais

Serves 6–8

Surprisingly, corn is not native to Italy or any other European country. It showed up in Italy through Veneto after America was discovered and widely known as granturco. As corn became more widely available, people began using it to make *polenta*.

This salad reflects both Italian and Middle Eastern influences by combining basil and cumin; evoking the essence of summer, it is a great accompaniment to any barbecue.

Ingredients

4 ears of corn, husk removed and brushed with olive oil

6–8 scallions, green part included, chopped

1 cup fresh basil, chopped

Juice of one large lemon

¼ cup olive oil

2 teaspoons cumin

Sea salt

Red pepper flakes

For the salad:

Preheat a gas or charcoal grill. Place the corn on the grill and roast until it gets some browning, but not overall.

Remove corn from grill and cool it completely.

Using a sharp knife, remove the corn kernels. In a medium bowl mix together the grilled corn, scallions, and basil.

For the dressing:

In a mixing bowl, mix the olive oil, cumin, and lemon juice; season with salt and red pepper flakes to taste. Add to the corn and mix well.

This salad can be eaten cold or at room temperature.

If there are leftovers, toss again before serving.

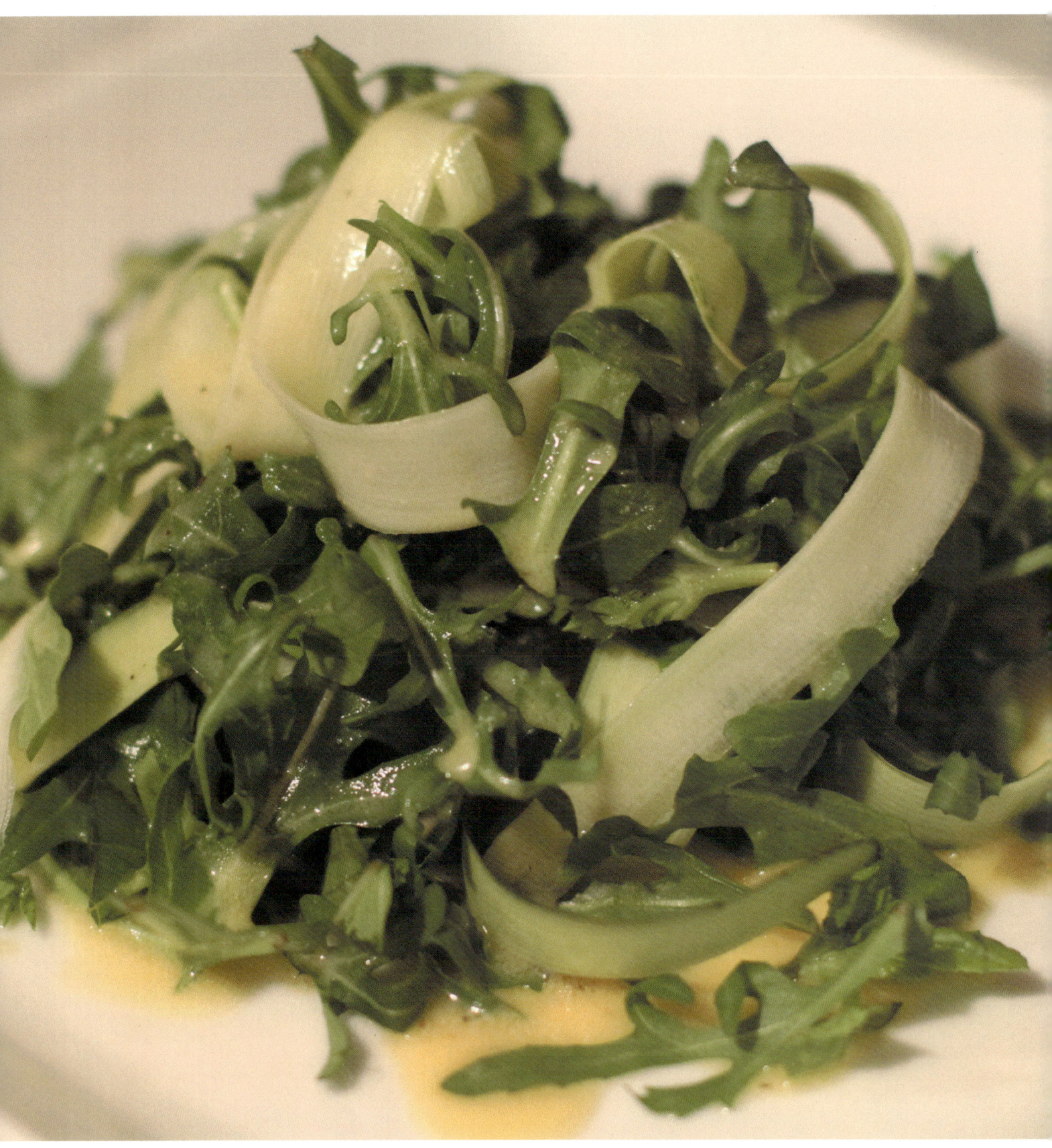

ZUCCHINI, BASIL AND ARUGULA SALAD

Insalata di Zuccini, Rucola, e Basilico

Serves 4–6

The Spanish explorers who came to the Americas brought back what they considered strange foods. Tomatoes, corn, peppers—as well as a family of melons—eventually found its way to Italy; once in Italy, this family of melons was named zucchini.

The native peoples of Mexico, as well as Central and South America, have been eating zucchini for centuries, but the zucchini we know today is a variety of summer squash developed in Italy, where it is eaten raw, stewed, or grilled.

Nonna Maria used to grow a variety called Cocozelle in her garden, which is shorter, plumper, and striped; she would simply slice it very thin and served it drizzled with extra virgin olive oil.

Ingredients

Juice of one lemon

5 tablespoons olive oil

1½ teaspoons Dijon mustard

½ teaspoon sugar

Sea salt and pepper

2 medium-size young zucchinis, sliced into very thin ribbons

1 small handful of basil leaves, chopped

1 large handful of arugula

Parmesan cheese ribbons using a vegetable peeler.

For the dressing:

Mix the lemon juice, olive oil, mustard, and sugar, whisking all ingredients in bowl to blend. Season with salt and pepper.

For the zucchini ribbons:

A simple vegetable peeler is all you'll need. Start by cutting off the ends of your zucchini; then, using your peeler, cut the strips lengthwise, stopping and turning when you see the seeds.

To assemble the salad:

Gently toss the zucchini strips, arugula, and basil with the dressing to coat. Make sure the salad is not overly dressed. Sprinkle the Parmesan cheese ribbons over the top of the salad, and serve immediately.

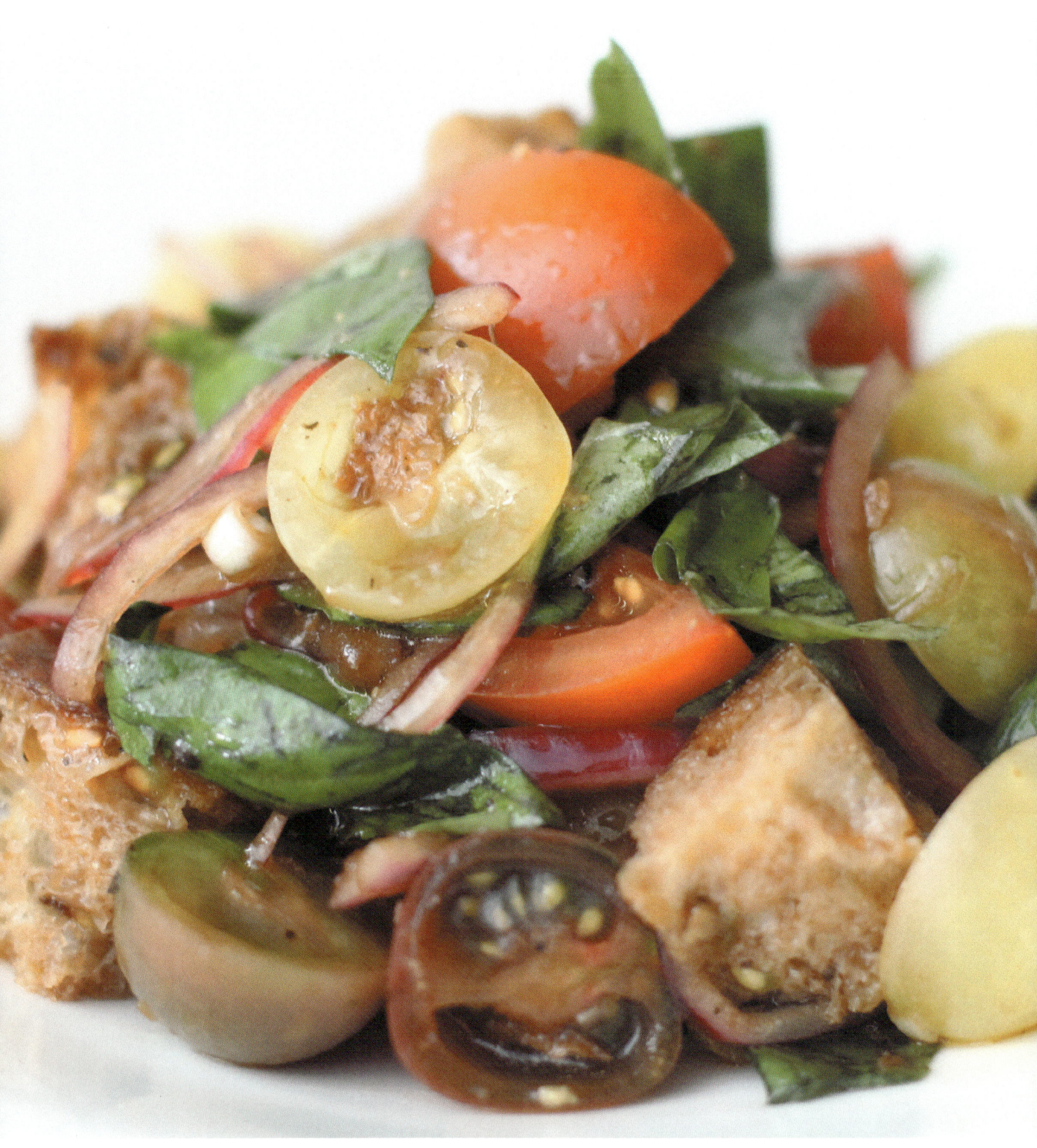

BREAD SALAD
Panzanella

Serves 4

Panzanella is a rustic dish, and a perfect example of the Cucina Povera. The original dish was developed by soaking stale bread in water, mixing it with vegetables from the garden. Tomatoes began appearing in this dish in the 16th century. This dish perpetuates the "nothing goes to waste mentality" that is an intrinsic part of Italian cooking and my own upbringing.

Ingredients

1 pound day-old country-style bread, crumbled or cut in 1–2" cubes (for a better presentation)

Extra virgin olive oil to taste

Balsamic vinegar or white wine vinegar to taste

Salt and pepper to taste

1 red onion, thinly sliced in half rounds

1 large spring basil, roughly chopped

4 ripe quartered tomatoes

½ cup of cold water

In a small bowl, mix the olive oil and vinegar, then season with enough salt and pepper.

Toss the dressing onto the bread, adding the roughly chopped basil leaves, tomatoes, and sliced onions until thoroughly combined. Let it sit until the bread has absorbed the vinegar and oil and has become moist. Some cold water may be added if bread it's too dry.

This salad develops a better taste and texture after letting it sit for an hour or two at room temperature. Serve drizzled with some extra virgin olive oil.

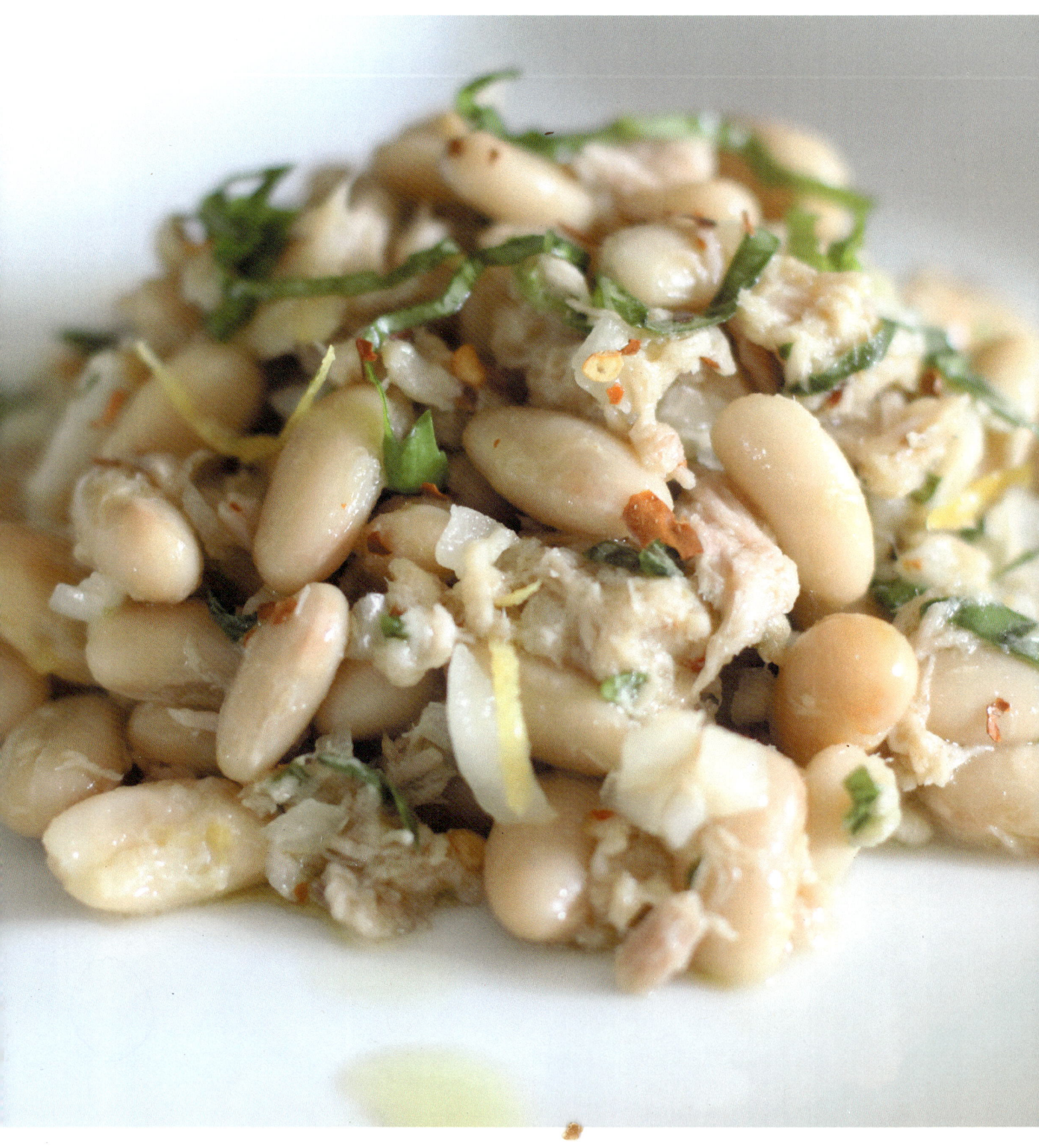

TUNA & CANNELLINI BEAN SALAD

Insalata Di Tonno E Fagioli

Serves 4

Tuna and white beans are a Tuscan classic—and a delicious one. This salad is good on its own as a side, or spooned over mixed greens or wilted spinach. The beauty of this recipe is that it can be tailored in many different ways depending on your tastes and what is in your kitchen. We used water-packed tuna and added our extra virgin olive oil of choice.

Ingredients

1 (5 ounces) can of tuna, drained

2 tablespoons extra virgin olive oil

Juice of 1 lemon

Red pepper flakes to taste

1 teaspoon dried oregano

½ small red or yellow onion, finely chopped

Handful of chopped fresh basil

1 (19 ounces) can of white cannellini beans, drained and rinsed

Salt to taste

Combine the tuna, olive oil, lemon juice, red pepper flakes, oregano, onion and basil. Gently mix the beans, being careful not to mash them.

Season with salt to taste, served by itself; you can also spoon it over crostini or a salad.

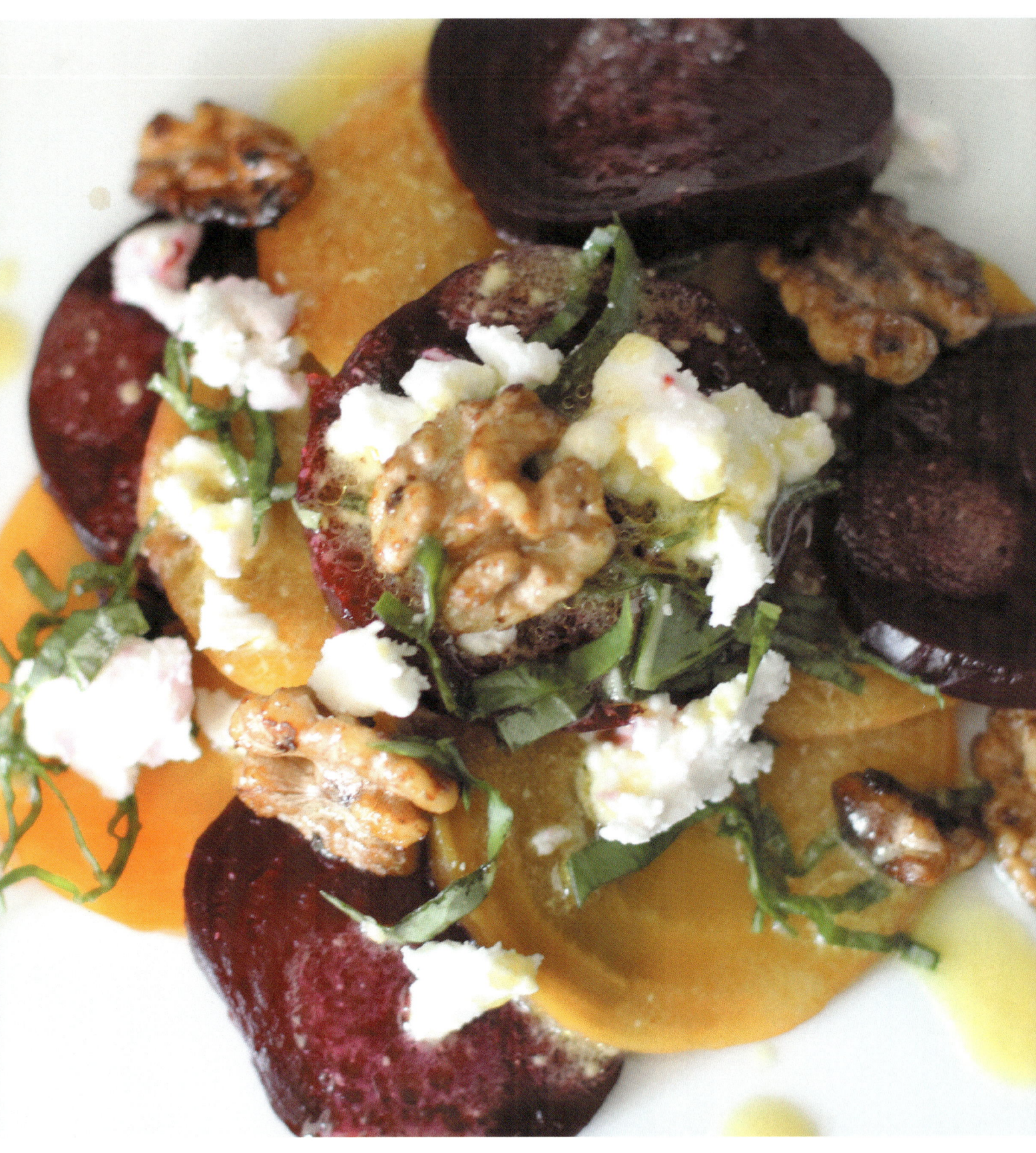

ROASTED BEET SALAD WITH GOAT CHEESE AND PECANS

Insalata Arrosto di Bietole con Formaggio di Capra e Noce

Serves 4–6

The best way to cook beets is to bake them; this releases an intense sweetness that no other cooking method can obtain. Red and golden beets make a great combination for this salad, which features a white balsamic vinegar and mustard dressing. Garnish with fresh basil chiffonade, chives or tarragon.

Ingredients

6 medium-size beets (3 red beets and 3 golden beets)

½ cup pecans

½ cup white balsamic vinegar

1 teaspoon Dijon mustard

4 tablespoons pure maple syrup or honey

¼ cup extra virgin olive oil plus 1 tablespoon for the pecans

8–10 fresh basil leaves (cut in ribbons)

Salt and pepper to taste

3 ounces crumbled goat cheese

While preparing ingredients, preheat oven to 400°F.

For the beets:

Remove the tops of the beets, wash and pat dry; wrap them individually in aluminum foil and bake for one hour or until done. They are done when they feel tender when prodded with a knife. Let them cool for about half an hour.

Peel and slice the beets in one-quarter-inch disc halves.

Cook the pecans in a skillet with a tablespoon of olive oil at medium heat for about two minutes. Add three tablespoons of maple syrup; remove from heat and season with sea salt and pepper.

For the dressing:

In a bowl, combine the vinegar, mustard, maple syrup, olive oil and basil until well combined; season with salt and pepper.

Gently cover the beets with the dressing and move to a plate. Sprinkle with the goat cheese and candied pecans.

Pour over the remaining dressing and serve.

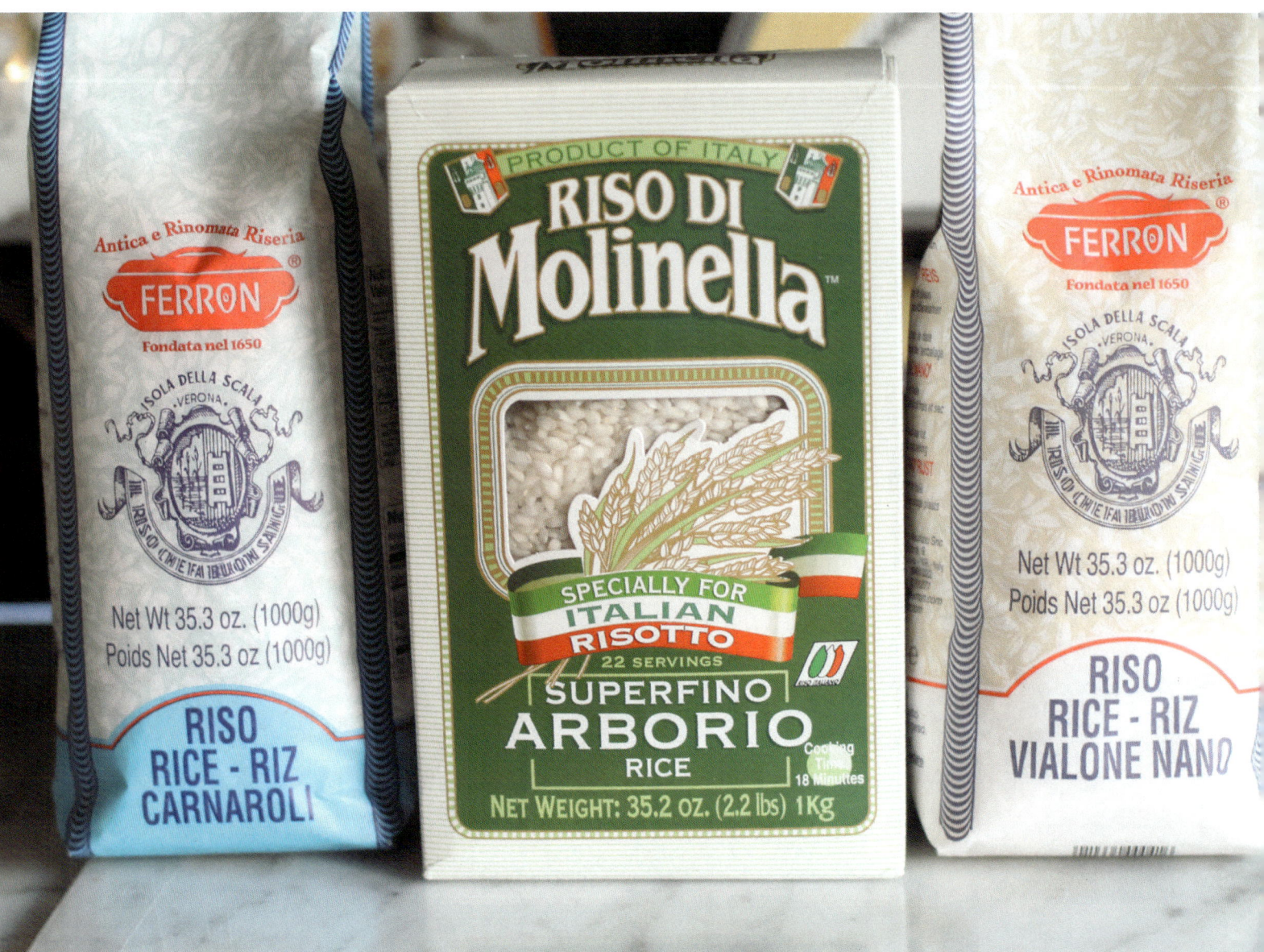

RISOTTO

Risotto: Northern Italian Decadence

There are few dishes as popular or as versatile as risotto. A northern Italian specialty, it is a warm rice dish and, contrary to what many think, very easy to make. This special type of rice is transformed into appetizers, side and main dishes, and even desserts.

The main type of rice used for risotto is a plump medium grain known as Arborio; two other hybrids are Carnaroli, which has a firm texture when cooked, and Vialone Nano, which has shorter grains that yield a less creamy sauce and take a little longer to cook.

The consumption of rice in Italy is more predominant in the north of the country and very small in comparison to pasta. Pasta is consumed mainly in the area known as Mezzogiorno, the regions south of Rome all the way to the end of the Italian peninsula and Sicily.

Risotto Styles

There are two basic styles of risotto; the main difference between the two of them is the consistency:

Venetian style—This style of risotto is known as *all'onda*. While you toss the risotto in the pan, the rice will rise up and break into peaks or waves. This is a very wet consistency.

Milanese style—The rice for risotto *alla Milanese* should be slightly moist and *al dente* when done. The consistency of this risotto is drier than the Venetian style, almost like a paella.

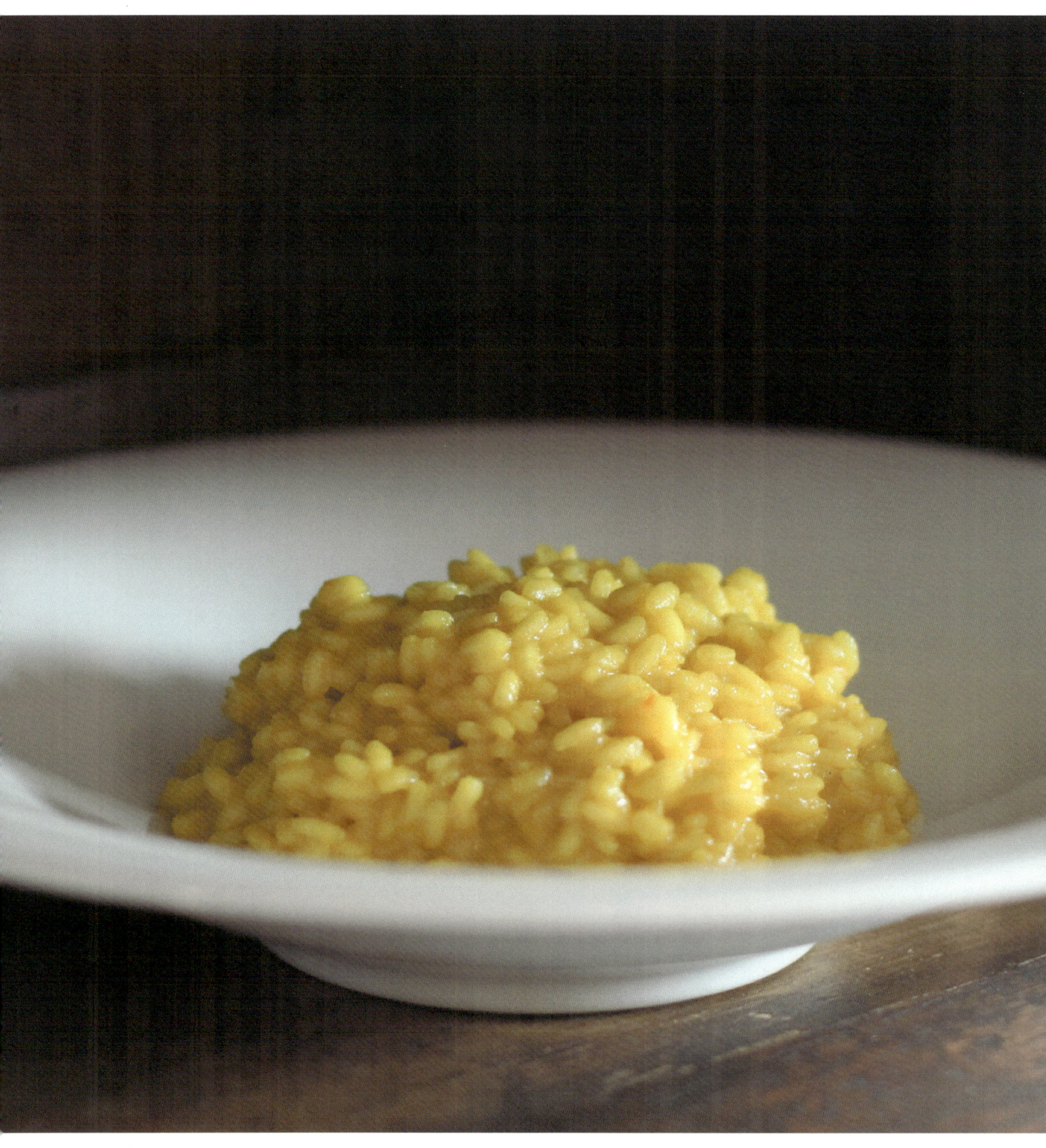

RISOTTO WITH SAFFRON, MILANESE STYLE

Risotto alla Milanese

This Milanese-style risotto is also popular in the Piedmont and Bologna regions. I omit the butter and cheese to let the delicate flavors of the saffron and rice speak for themselves. The creamy consistency comes from the high amount of starch in this type of rice. Arborio rice is the most frequently used as well as Vialone Nano and Carnaroli.

Ingredients

5–6 cups hot chicken broth, more as needed

5 tablespoons olive oil

1 medium yellow onion, finely chopped

2 cups Arborio rice

½ cup dry white wine

½ teaspoon saffron threads

½ cup grated Parmesan cheese
(optional: 1 tablespoon extra virgin olive oil may be used instead)

Salt and freshly ground black pepper to taste

In a medium-size pot, bring the stock to a boil; reduce the heat to low and keep it at a low simmer.

In a medium-size pan, and over gentle heat, warm the olive oil and add the finely chopped onion. Cook until translucent.

Next, add the Arborio rice, gently stirring to coat all the rice grains. Cook for two to three minutes. A white spot will appear in the middle of the grains; when that occurs, add the white wine. Gently simmer until the wine has evaporated.

Next, add a small quantity of the stock and season with salt to taste. While still simmering, gently stir the risotto, and continue to do so until almost all the liquid has evaporated. (Don't boil it dry, though!) Once almost dry, add another small quantity of stock, and repeat the process. You will need to continue to do this for around 15–18 minutes. Taste the rice and check for "bite" before adding the next quantity of stock.

Add the saffron, then add more stock; stir and taste for your preferred level of salt. Continue stirring the risotto—at this point the rice should be creamy, making it a good time to check for doneness.

When fully cooked, add the olive oil and stir; place a lid on the pan and remove from the heat. Let the risotto sit for two to three minutes, and serve immediately.

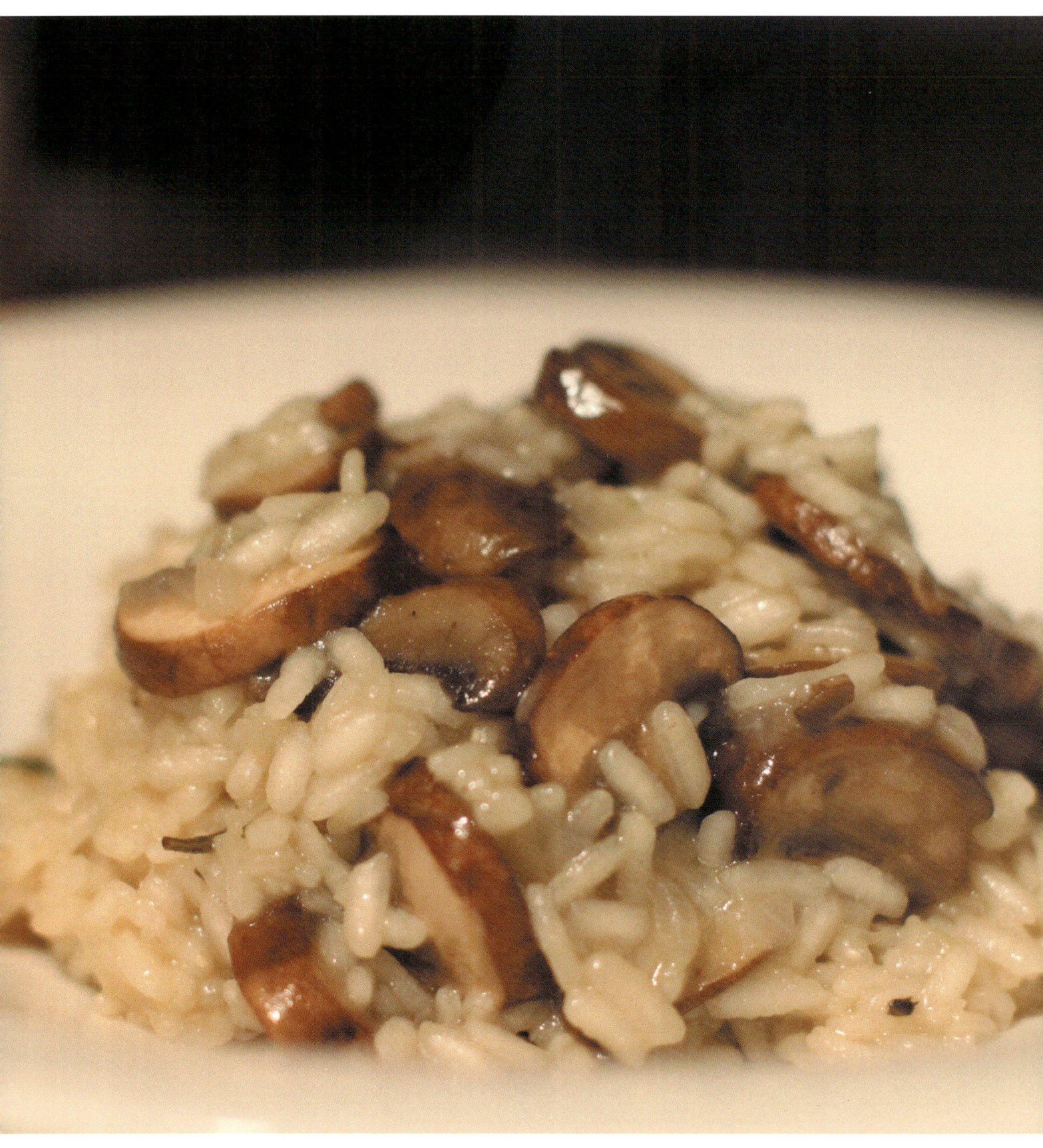

MUSHROOM RISOTTO
Risotto ai Funghi

Porcini is the traditional type of mushroom used in risotto and are much sought-after for their musky flavor and aroma. Mushroom risotto is one of our favorite dishes, and autumn is the best time to make it as a side dish for roasted meats or poultry. We use the most common and readily available cremini or white mushrooms, which are milder in flavor but nevertheless delicious.

The Milanese prefer to use Carnaroli rice for their risotto recipes, since they tend to be of a drier consistency (as found in Spanish paella) whereas Vialone Nano is the type commonly used in Veneto. Instead of finishing the risotto with cheese or butter, we drizzle it with extra virgin olive oil. Cheese and butter tends to overpower the delicate flavors.

Ingredients

5–6 cups reduced-sodium chicken broth

4 tablespoons of extra virgin olive oil, plus some for drizzling

3 cups of fresh cremini mushrooms, trimmed and thinly sliced

1½ teaspoon of fresh rosemary, finely chopped

1 medium yellow onion, finely chopped (1 cup)

1 pound of Arborio rice

½ cup dry white wine

In a medium-size sauce pot, bring the stock to a simmer, and let it continue simmering at a very low heat.

In a medium-size sauté pan, heat two tablespoons of olive oil over medium heat. Sauté the mushrooms with the rosemary, and season with salt and pepper. Cook until the mushrooms have released their water and a sauce has formed, approximately 10 minutes. Remove from heat and set aside.

Heat the remaining two tablespoons of olive oil in a large heavy pot over medium-high heat and sauté the chopped onion, stirring until just translucent, about five minutes. Add rice and cook, stirring, for one minute. Add the white wine and cook, stirring until absorbed, for about one minute.

Stir one cup of simmering broth into rice and cook, stirring constantly, keeping it at a strong simmer until absorbed. This whole process will take about 25 minutes. Continue cooking and adding broth, about one cup at a time, stirring frequently while allowing each addition be absorbed before adding the next. Repeat until rice becomes tender and creamy looking. Add the cooked mushrooms with their juice, and combine well until the rice is al dente. Thin with some of remaining broth if the rice has become too dry.

Remove from heat. Finish the risotto with some extra virgin olive oil and mix well.

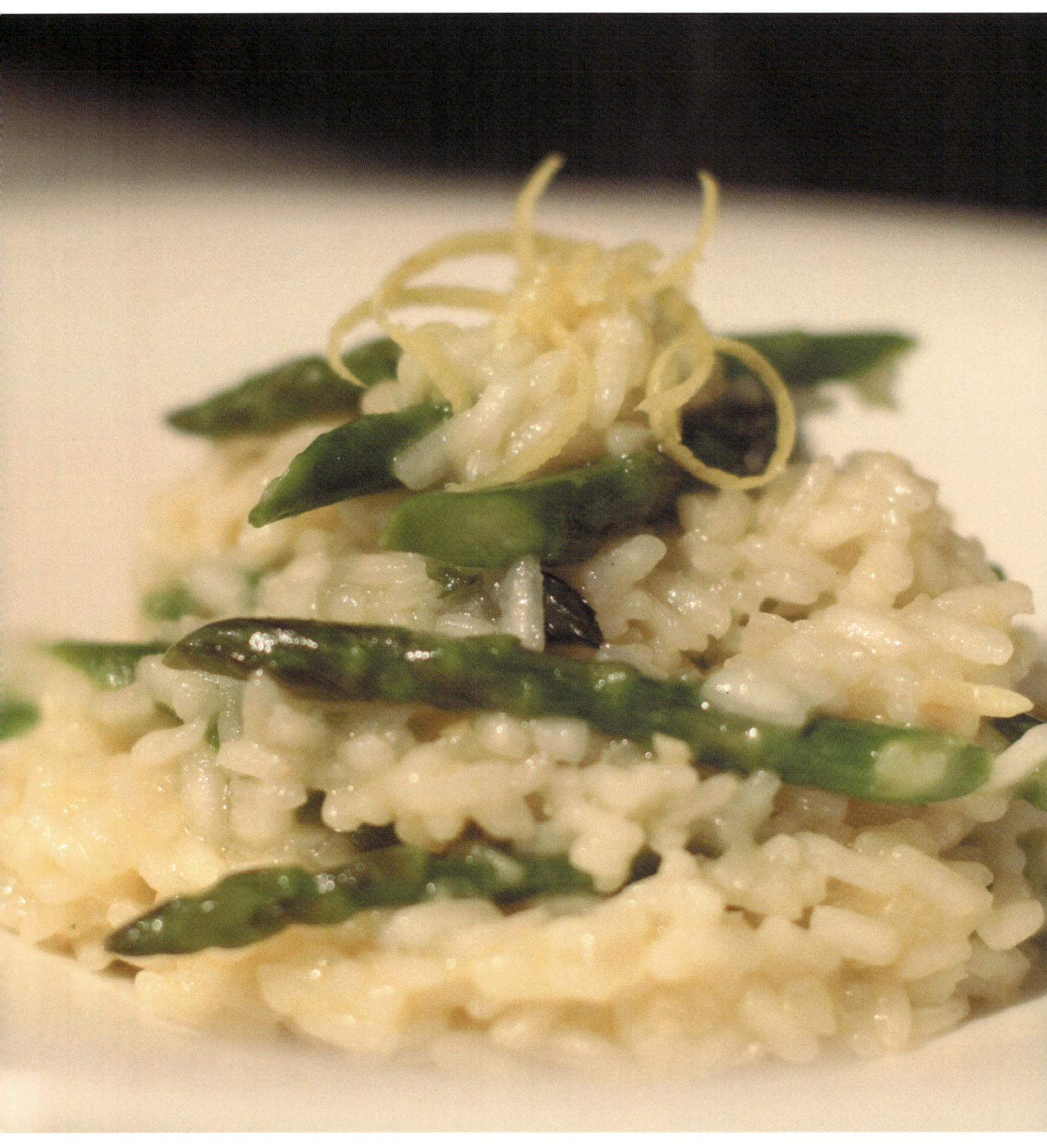

RISOTTO WITH CHICKEN, ASPARAGUS AND LEMON

Risotto con Pollo, Esparagi e Limone

In the middle ages, Northern Italy was the main producer of asparagus, which was considered a luxury in that time. A recipe from the Renaissance calls for the spears to be boiled for a few minutes and served as a side dish with a splash of olive oil and lemon juice, or served with hot with melted butter and Parmesan.

This springtime risotto showcases the herbaceous asparagus flavor with lemon and chicken.

Ingredients

5–6 cups chicken broth

4 tablespoons olive oil

1 chicken breast, skinless and boned, cut in one-inch cubes

1½ cups Arborio Rice

1 medium-size onion, finely chopped

½ cup white wine

1 pound asparagus cut into 1½ inch pieces

Zest of 2 large lemons

¼ cup fresh parsley, finely chopped

Sea salt and pepper

In a medium-size pot, bring the stock to a boil. Reduce the heat to low and keep it at a low simmer.

In a medium-size pan, over medium heat, add two tablespoons of olive oil. Add the chicken and partially cook for about five minutes; stir and season with salt and pepper. Chicken will be only partially cooked; remove from pan and keep warm.

Add the remaining two tablespoons of olive oil; at medium heat, begin cooking the onion until translucent, about 8-10 minutes.

Add the Arborio rice, gently stirring to coat all the rice grains. Cook for around 2–3 minutes until a white spot appears in the middle of the grains; add the white wine. Gently simmer until the wine has evaporated. Add a small quantity of the stock, and season with salt to taste. While still simmering, gently stir the risotto, and continue to do so until almost all the liquid has evaporated. (Don't boil it dry, though!) Once almost dry, add another small quantity of stock, and repeat the process. Repeat for 15–18 minutes. Taste the rice and check for "bite" before adding the next quantity of stock. After 15–18 minutes, add the chicken, and continue stirring and adding stock.

Stir the asparagus and lemon zest into the risotto and taste for your preferred level of salt. Continue stirring the risotto; at this point the rice should be creamy. Check for doneness of the rice and chicken.When rice is cooked and chicken has cooked completely, you can add the Parmesan cheese and parsley. Stir, place a lid on the pan, and remove from the heat. Let the risotto sit for two to three minutes and serve immediately.

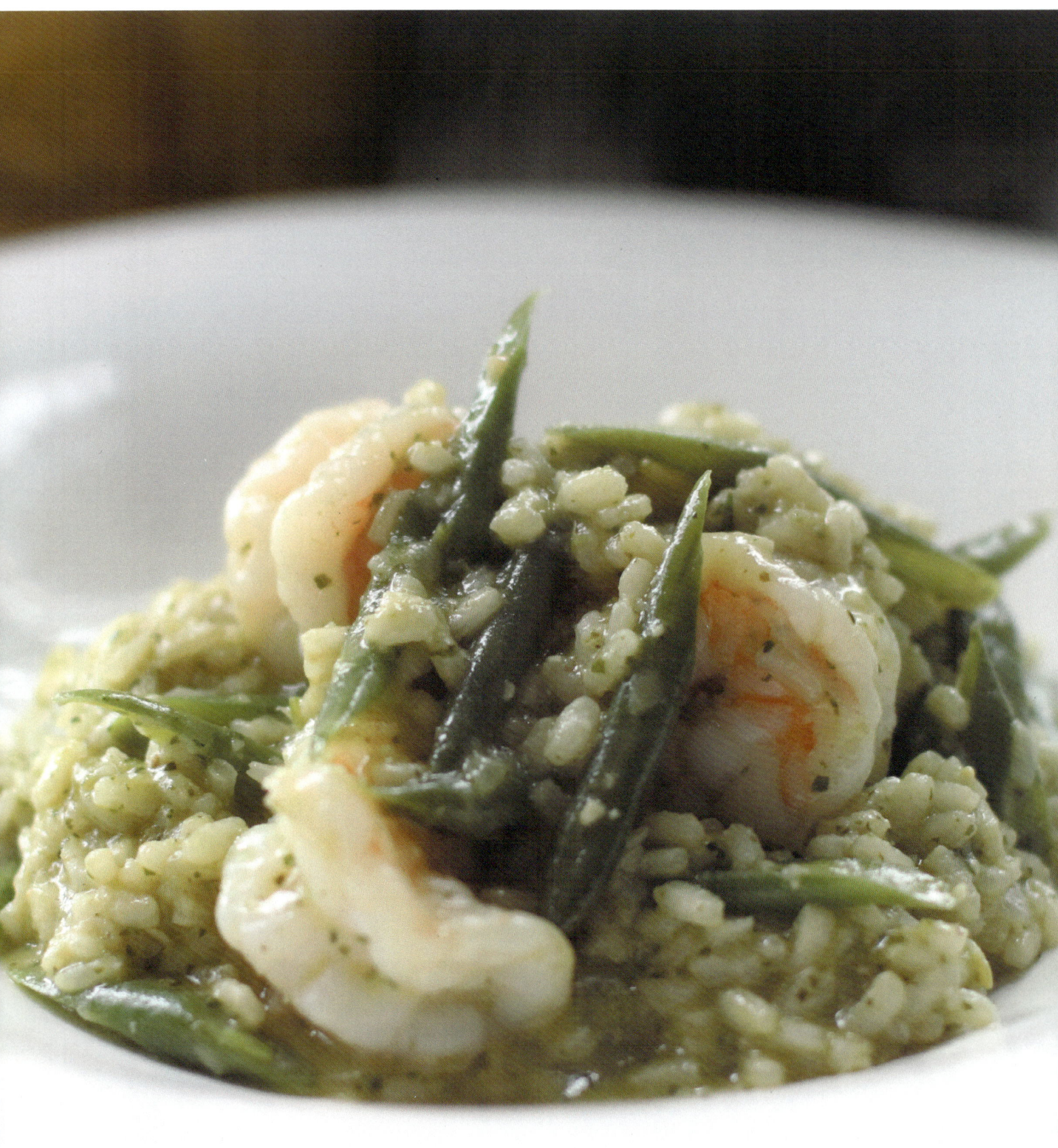

RISOTTO WITH SHRIMP, STRING BEANS, AND PESTO

Risotto con Scampi, Fagiolini e Pesto

We make our own fresh pesto for this recipe, but if you are short of time, you can use store-bought pesto. To make your own, follow our simple yet delicious recipe on page 3.

Ingredients

5 to 6 cups chicken stock

5 tablespoons extra virgin olive oil

1 pound large shrimp, uncooked, peeled, deveined

1 cup fresh string beans, cut into one-inch diagonal pieces

1 medium yellow onion, finely chopped

¼ cup white wine

1½ cups Arborio rice

½ cup pesto

Sea salt

Freshly ground black pepper

Bring stock to simmer in medium saucepan. Reduce heat; keep simmering.

Heat two tablespoons of olive oil in medium skillet over medium heat. Add the shrimp and string beans. Sauté for about two minutes until shrimp begin to turn pink. Set aside.

Heat the remaining three tablespoons of olive oil in heavy large saucepan over medium heat. Add onion and sauté until onion is translucent, about four minutes. Add rice and stir to coat, about two minutes.

Add the wine and cook until alcohol has evaporated; then add one cup of stock, stirring often until mostly absorbed.

Continue adding stock mixture one cup at a time. Stir often and simmer until liquid is absorbed before adding more; repeat for about 20 minutes.

Stir in reserved shrimp and string beans with their cooking liquid; add the pesto, combine well, and continue stirring just until rice is tender and mixture is creamy (about five minutes longer). Remove from heat and serve immediately.

SOUPS

Zuppe

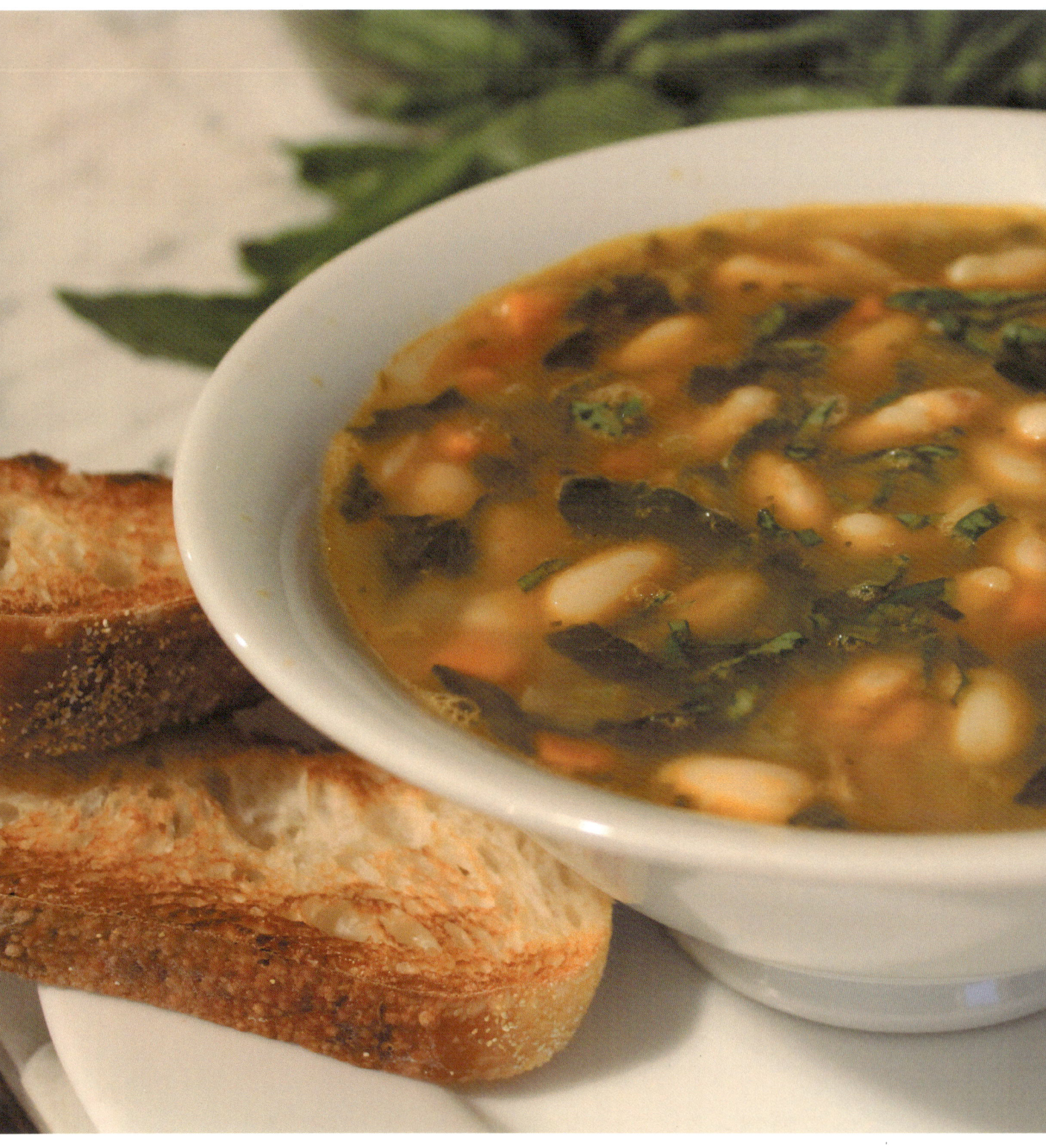

TUSCAN RIBOLLITA SOUP
Ribollita Toscana

La Ribollita, a main dish of Tuscan cuisine (also known as Minestra di Pane), is the perfect soup for fall or winter. Filled with vegetables such as Cavolo Nero (kale) and legumes such as cannellini beans, it is enriched with slices of stale Tuscan unsalted bread instead of meat. It all starts with the *battuto* or *soffritto*, which is basically an Italian term for finely chopped aromatics.

As a true Tuscan peasant dish, there is no exact measuring or perfect dicing. Usually it starts with double the amount of onions to every other ingredient. There really are no rules on this; use your own palate or what's available to create the combination you like.

Though there are different types of kale, the most common types are the curly kale and black or Lacinato Tuscan kale. Curly kale ranges from light green to purple, and is one of the more bitter types.

The kale leaves will retain a firm texture even after cooked for a long time. We prefer to serve the bread *alongside* the soup rather than *in* the soup, in order to obtain a less dense and heavy soup.

Ingredients

5 tablespoons extra virgin olive oil

1 large yellow onion, finely chopped

1 garlic clove, minced

½ cup minced Italian parsley

3 large carrots, finely chopped

3 celery stalks, finely chopped

1 quart (32 ounces) chicken broth

½ cup chopped tomatoes (canned)

2 cans (15 ounces each) cannellini beans, drained and rinsed

3 cups chopped black kale, rinsed and stems removed

Slices of Tuscan or any rustic style of bread, toasted

Place ¼ cup of the olive oil in a deep, heavy-bottomed saucepan or pot (cast iron or enameled cast iron work well).

Add the onions, garlic, parsley, carrots, and celery to the pot. Stir and season with the salt and pepper.

Cook over medium heat for 20 minutes, stirring often; add the chicken broth, tomatoes, half of the beans, and cook for another 15–20 minutes.

Add the kale and remaining beans, and cook for another 15 minutes. Remove from heat; serve hot, sprinkled with cheese, and with toasted slices of bread on the side.

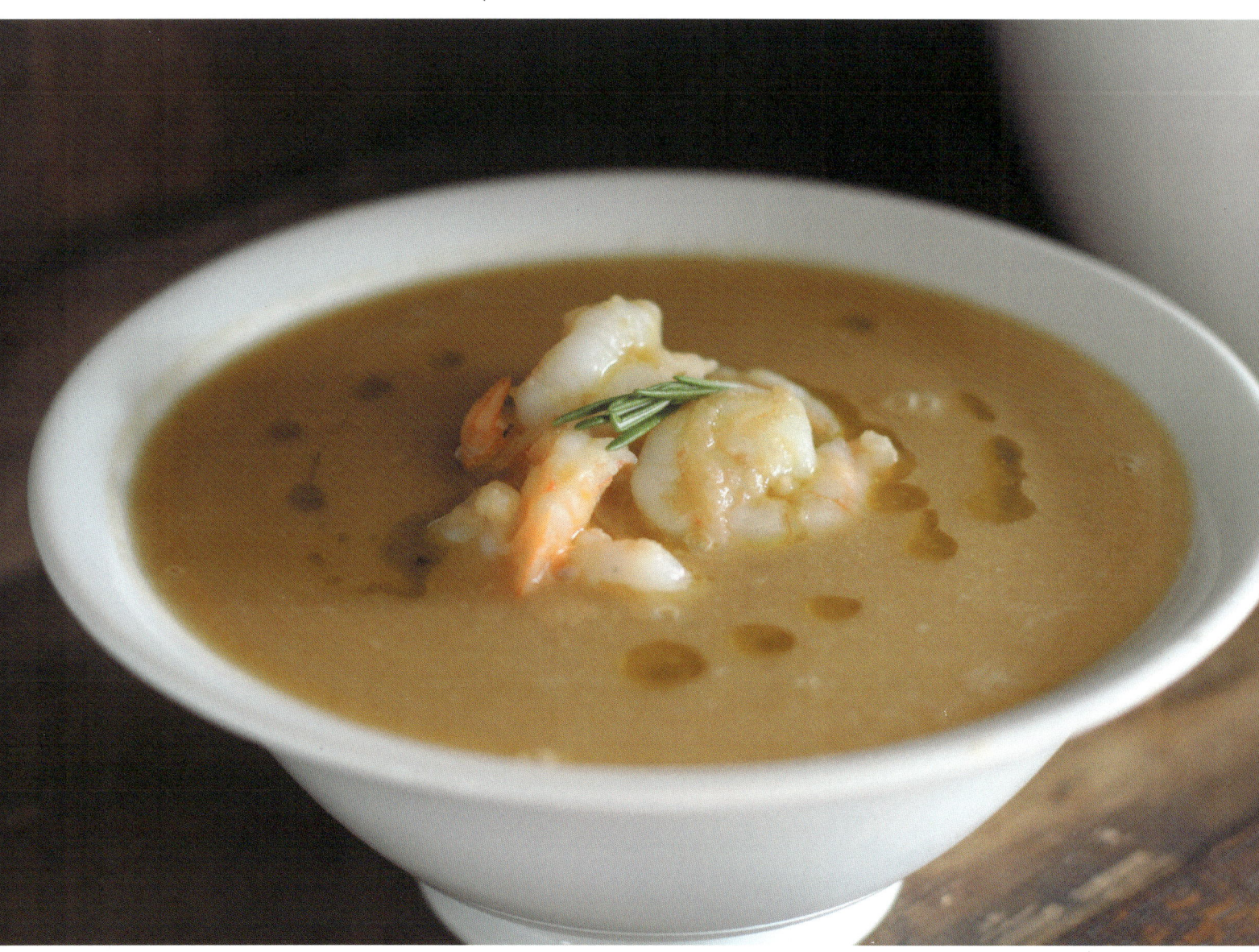

CHICKPEA SOUP WITH SHRIMP

Minestra di Ceci e Gambieri

While I was homeschooled in Fiesole, chickpeas were used heavily during the Holy Week when the family observed the strict fish diet for all seven days. Chickpeas—popular in Spain and Portugal during the Arab occupation and widespread during Roman times—were cooked into dry fish stew with tomatoes, soups, and into a thin bread called *torta di ceci*, or *cecina*—an unleavened flat bread of chickpea flour originating in Genoa (see recipe on Page 17). In Tuscany, where it is called cecina, it is served stuffed into small focaccia (mainly in Pisa) or between two slices of bread, and is a traditional inexpensive street food in Livorno. It is sold in pizzerias and bakeries in many towns.

This soup is quick and hearty, and the addition of shrimp sautéed with rosemary brings this humble soup to yet another level.

Ingredients

5–6 tablespoons of extra virgin olive oil

1 small onion, finely chopped

1 small spring of fresh rosemary, finely chopped

3 cans of chickpeas, rinsed and drained

½ cup chopped canned tomatoes

3–4 cups low-sodium chicken broth

8–12 medium-size shrimp, shell removed and deveined

Sea salt

Freshly ground black pepper

In a large pan, heat two tablespoons of olive oil at medium heat; stir the onion and half of the rosemary (about one teaspoon) and cook until the onion is translucent. Add the chickpeas and tomatoes and cook for about eight to ten minutes. Add some broth, remove from heat, and let it cool once you've set it aside.

When chickpeas are cool enough to handle, pour them into a blender or food processor and purée until smooth (or chunky, if desired).

In a large soup pot, stir in the puréed chickpeas and remaining stock. Season with salt and pepper and bring to a gentle simmer for about 15–20 minutes. You can add water or stock to thin the consistency of the soup, if you wish.

While the soup simmers, heat the remaining olive oil in a frying pan over medium heat. Add the remaining rosemary and shrimp; season with sea salt and cook until done.

Serve the soup and garnish with some shrimp and a drizzle of the olive oil used to cook the shrimp.

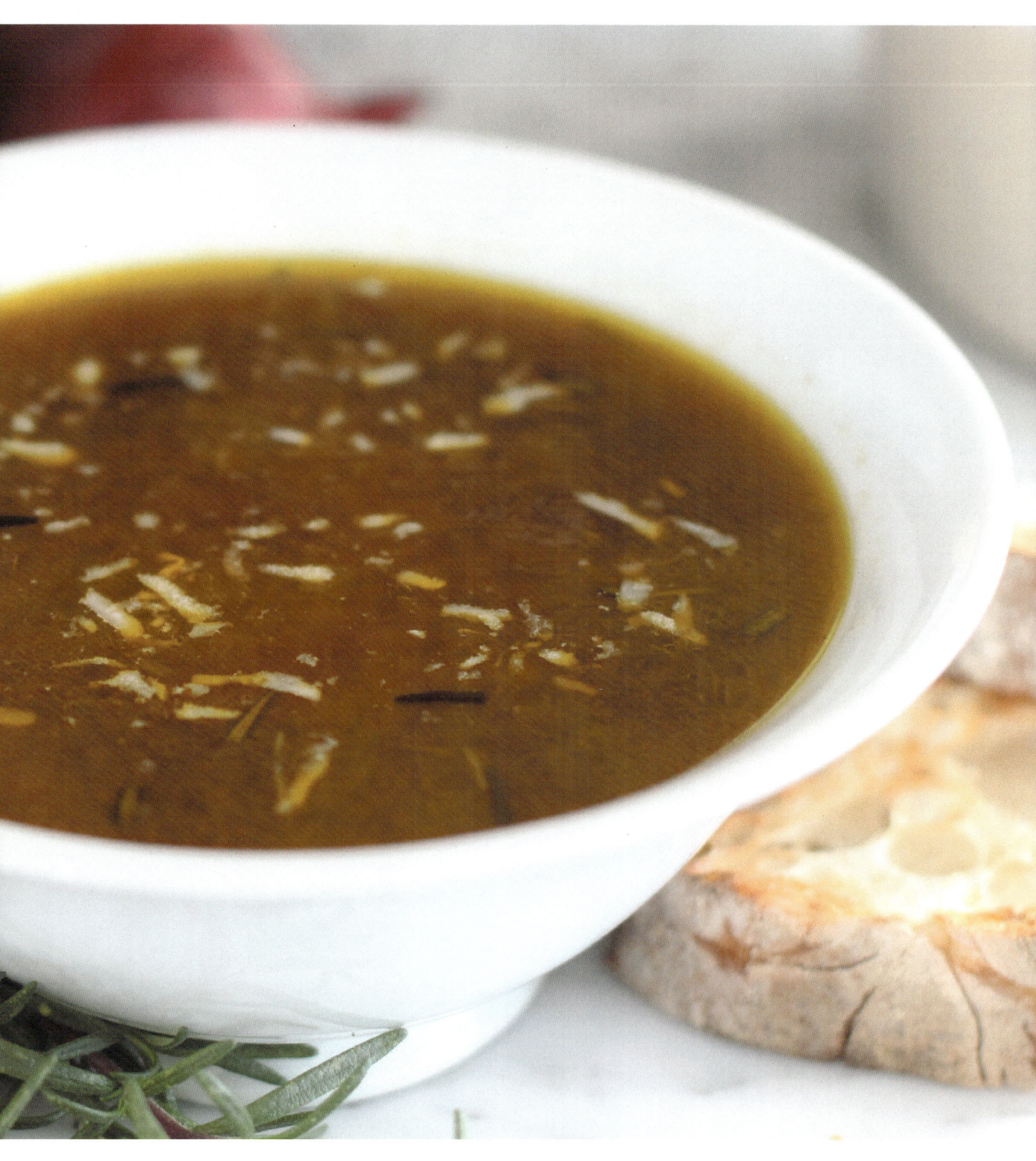

TUSCAN RED ONION SOUP
Carabaccia

Serves 4–6

This is another soup that originated in the Middle Ages. Catarina de' Medici was so fond of this soup she brought it with her when she married Henry II of France. Once in France, this evolved into the well-known French onion soup.

Ingredients

½ cup extra virgin olive oil

1 sprig fresh rosemary, finely chopped, approximately 1 tablespoon if dry

2 pounds red onions, very thinly sliced.

7 cups chicken or beef stock

Sea salt and black pepper to taste

1 cup grated Parmesan or pecorino cheese

Country-style bread, sliced and toasted

In a large soup pot, heat the olive oil over medium heat. Add the rosemary and onions and cook for 25–30 minutes, stirring occasionally until the onions are caramelized. Add the stock, season with salt and pepper, and cook for another 30 minutes.

When done, dust the soup with the cheese and serve with the toasted bread.

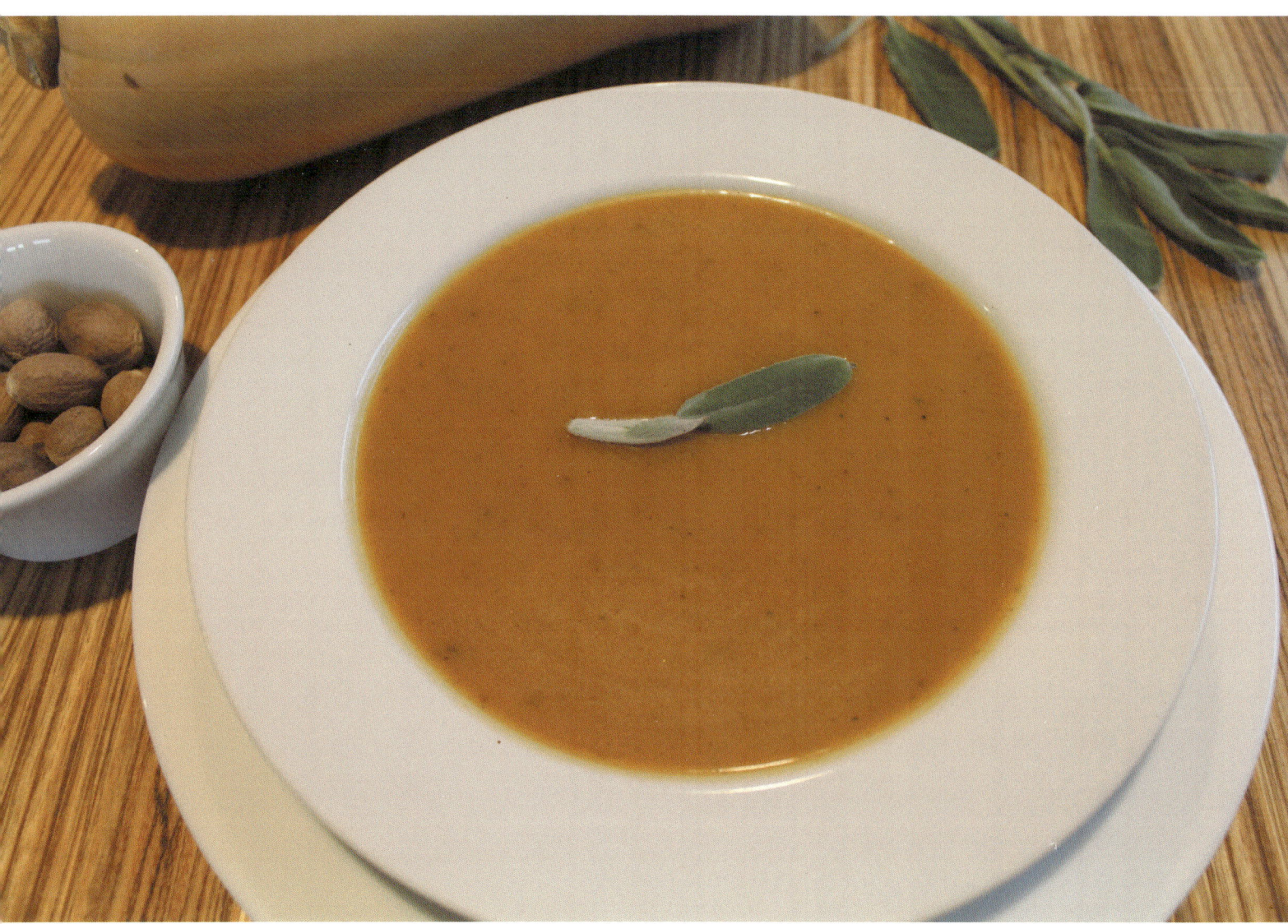

CREAMY BUTTERNUT PUMPKIN SOUP WITH SAGE

Crema di Zucca con Salvia

Serves 4–6

In Italy, the butternut squash is referred to as pumpkin. It is a versatile vegetable—and technically, a fruit. Italians use pumpkin in many dishes, including, risottos, soups, breads, cakes, puddings, and flans. It can be roasted or puréed. We like to use butternut squash for this soup as it has sweet flesh and great color. Always choose fresh, never canned. This soup is easy to make and is good for all occasions.

Ingredients

3 pounds butternut squash, peeled, seeded and cut into one-inch chunks

4 tablespoons extra virgin olive oil

1 large garlic clove, finely chopped

8–10 medium-size sage leaves, finely chopped

Salt and pepper

1 medium-size yellow onion, roughly chopped

3 cups chicken stock

¼ teaspoon nutmeg

¼ teaspoon cinnamon

Water to thin (optional)

Milk to thicken (optional)

Preheat oven to 375°F.

Put the chunks of butternut squash in a roasting pan. Toss it with two tablespoons of olive oil, adding garlic, sage, and salt and pepper. Place the roasting pan in the oven and cook for 35–45 minutes, or until the flesh is completely tender and golden. Pull from the oven and set aside when done.

While the squash is in the oven, heat up the remaining two tablespoons of olive oil in a heavy, broad-bottomed saucepan or pot and add the chopped onion. Sauté at medium heat for about 10 minutes, until the onions are translucent.

Add the squash to the onion. Pour in the stock, cinnamon, nutmeg, season with salt and pepper, and bring to the boil. Simmer for about 20 minutes, then let the soup cool.

Purée in a blender and check the seasoning by tasting. Bring back to the pot and adjust the thickness of the soup to your own taste by adding water to thin or milk to thicken.

ENTRÉES

Primo Piatto

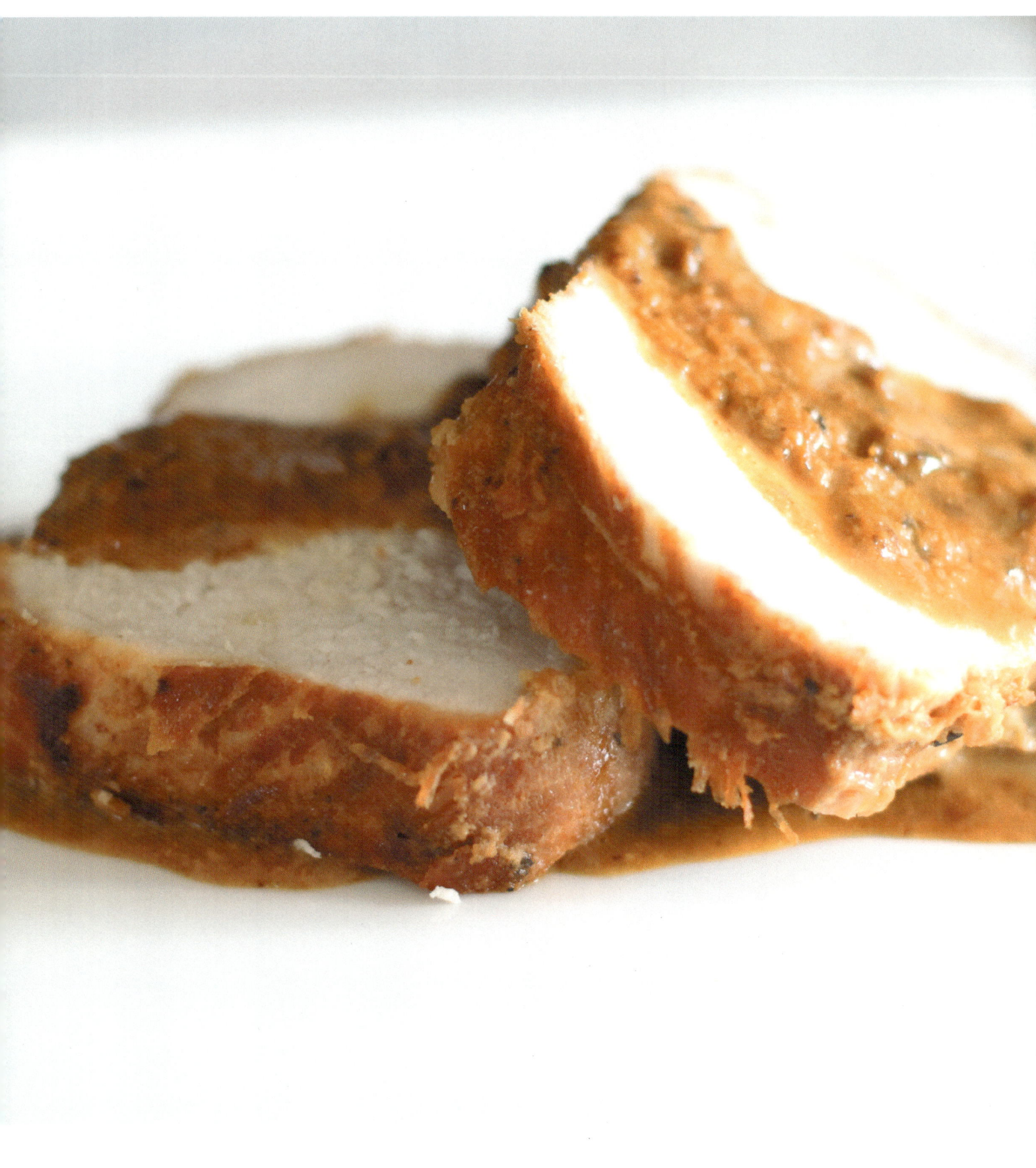

PORK TENDERLOIN BRAISED IN MILK, BOLOGNESE STYLE

Maiale al Latte

Serves 4–6

As strange as it may seem to the American palate, cooking meat in milk is a traditional and very common technique used throughout northern Italy, especially in Parma and Bologna.

The milk's lactic acid acts as an effective tenderizer, and the milk itself becomes a delicious golden, nutty sauce. It may not look like the most elegant dish as the milk curdles, turning into a grainy or ricotta-like substance.

There are several versions: some include prosciutto, garlic, and herbs, but lemon zest seems to prevail throughout all those versions.

Ingredients

4 pounds boned pork loin

2 cloves garlic, slivered

1 teaspoon lemon zest

2½ cups whole milk, plus more as needed
     for sauce

2 tablespoons olive oil

Sea salt and pepper

1 ½ teaspoon of rosemary, chopped if fresh

Tie the meat with cooking twine so it will hold its shape; dust with salt and pepper.

Heat the oil in a pot and brown the meat on all sides, then add the garlic. Cook for one minute, add the lemon zest, and pour the milk over everything. Reduce the heat and simmer uncovered until the pork is done (60–90 minutes). While simmering, turn the meat occasionally, scraping the bottom of the pot to keep the curds (which form as a result of the interaction between lemon and milk) from sticking.

By the time the pork is done, almost all the liquid should have evaporated; at this point, stir the curds often to prevent them from burning. Add more milk, enough to make sauce.

Let the roast sit for a few minutes; slice it finely, spoon the curds over the slices, and serve.

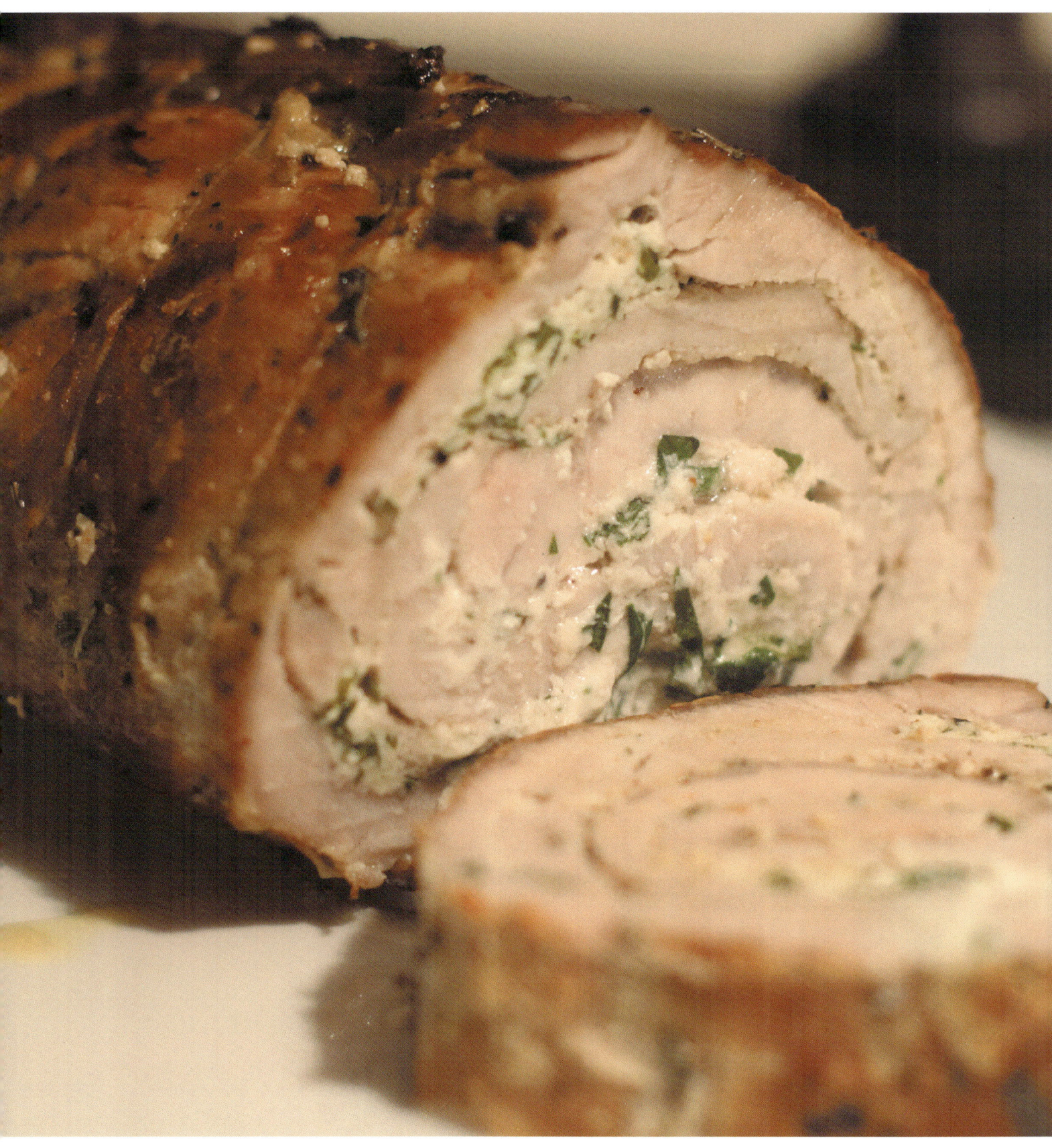

PORK LOIN STUFFED WITH RICOTTA AND SPINACH

Involtini di Maiale

Serves 4

Ricotta, spinach, and nutmeg add flavor and moisture to a leaner cut such as pork tenderloin, which many times can be overcooked and turn into a overly dry piece of meat. We use prosciutto to wrap the loin to add extra flavor and crunchiness, but it can be omitted, if you wish.

Ingredients

3 or 4 pounds of pork loin, butterflied (slice it in half lengthwise almost all the way through)

3 tablespoons extra virgin olive oil

2 cloves garlic, finely minced

1 (9–10 ounces) bag of fresh spinach, or 2 large bunches, trimmed and washed

Sea salt to taste

Black pepper to taste

1 cup ricotta cheese

½ teaspoon of freshly ground nutmeg

1 sprig rosemary, finely chopped

Optional: 1 (4 ounces) package of prosciutto

Pre-heat oven to 375°F.

To butterfly the loin, arrange it on a work surface with short end facing you. Holding the knife parallel to work surface and beginning along one long side, cut about half an inch above the underside of roast. Continue slicing inward, pulling back the meat with your free hand and unrolling the roast like a carpet.

In a large, deep, nonstick pan or pot, heat two tablespoons of olive oil. Add garlic and sauté for one minute. Add all spinach, salt, and pepper, and toss with garlic and oil. Cover pan and cook on low for about one minute. Uncover pan, turn the heat on high, and cook spinach for another minute or two, stirring with a wooden spoon until all the spinach is wilted. Using a slotted spoon, lift the spinach into a sieve; squeeze and let it drain. Gently squeeze one more time; transfer to a cutting board and chop, then set aside.

In a mixing bowl, combine the ricotta with the spinach and nutmeg, and season with salt and pepper.

Spread the ricotta mix over the butterfly pork loin and slowly roll up into a cylinder. Roll up the pork loin into a compact cylinder and tie it with kitchen twine at two-inch intervals. Season the pork loin with the chopped rosemary, sea salt, and freshly ground pepper.

Place the loin in a roasting pan, cover with aluminum foil, and bake for 45–50 minutes; remove the foil and continue roasting for another 15 minutes until a golden crust has formed.

Prosciutto option:

Before tying the loin, you can lay the prosciutto slices crosswise over the loin, overlapping slightly. Tuck the ends of the prosciutto underneath the loin, and tie it with kitchen twine at two-inch intervals.

Place the loin in a roasting pan, cover with aluminum foil, and bake for 40–45 minutes; remove the foil and continue roasting for another 15 minutes until a golden crust has formed.

Untie the pork loin and carve the meat into thick slices.

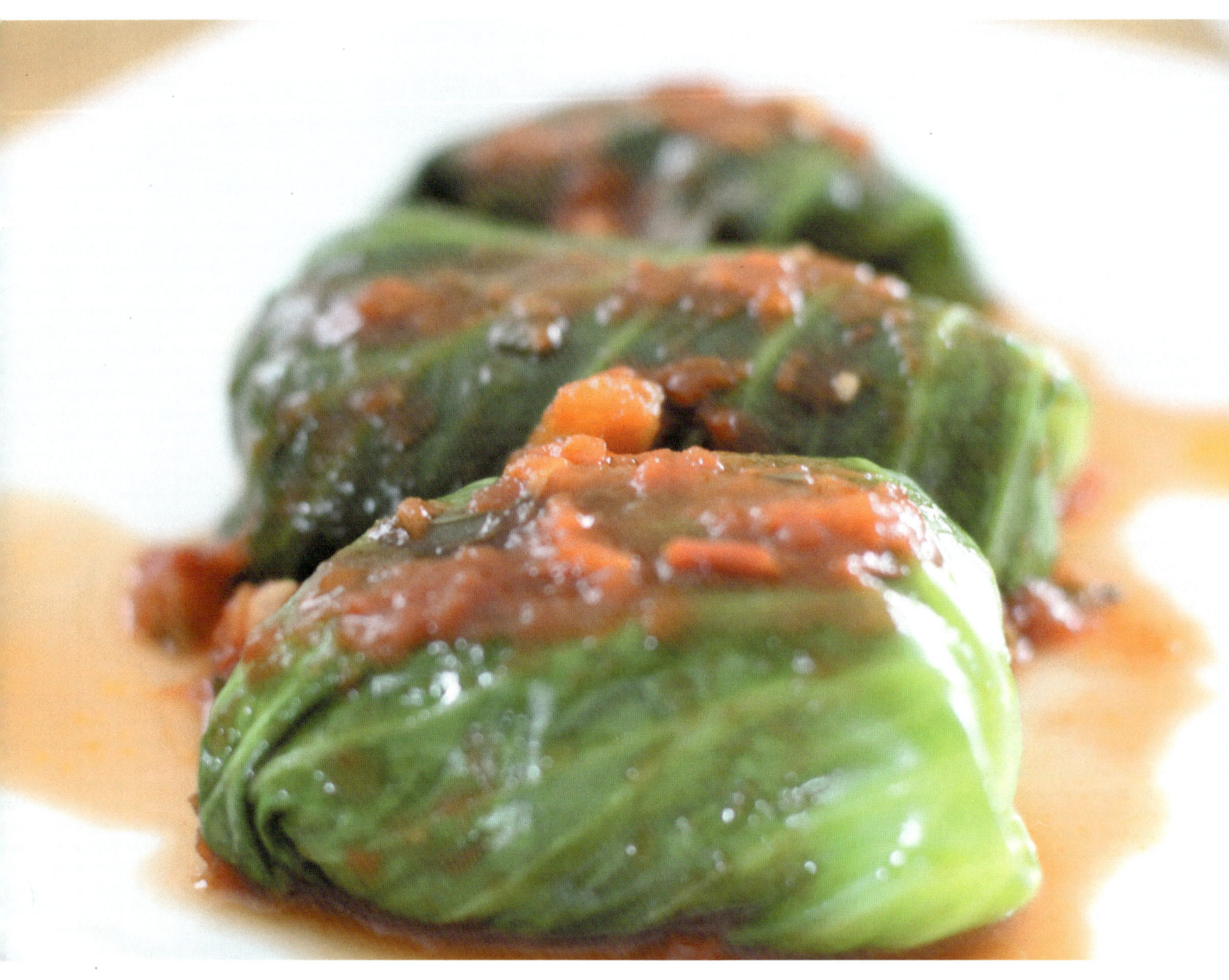

Savoy cabbage is sweeter, more tender, and lacks the sulphuric odor of the more commonly used green cabbage.

STUFFED SAVOY CABBAGE PARCELS WITH PORK IN A TOMATO-BASIL SAUCE

Fagottini di Verza con Salsa di Pomodoro e Basilico

Serves 4-5

This recipe traces its origins back to the 18th century when it was served with stock; the tomato sauce is a 19th century addition. While studying in Italy, I noticed that they never added rice or bread to their meat stuffing. This was rather a more common addition made by Italian-Americans who needed to increase the volume of their food in the early 1900s when, as new arrivals to the country, food was expensive and not the best quality.

Ingredients

2 large cloves garlic, finely minced

4 tablespoons olive oil

2 medium-size springs of fresh rosemary, minced

Red pepper flakes

1 (46 ounces) can crushed tomatoes

2 cups chicken stock

1 cup shredded fresh basil

1 large Savoy cabbage

1½ pounds pork loin, cut in small two-inch pieces

1 large yellow onion, finely minced

½ cup chopped celery

½ cup grated Parmesan cheese

¼ teaspoon grated nutmeg

This recipe is divided into three easy steps: a simple 20 minute tomato sauce, the sautéed pork filling, and the assembling of the parcels.

For the sauce: In a large saucepan, over medium heat, sauté one chopped clove of garlic in one tablespoon of olive oil; do not let it brown. Add half of the rosemary and red pepper flakes to taste. Add the crushed tomatoes, one cup of stock, and half of the chopped basil. Season with salt, and cook for 15 minutes. Keep warm when working on the cabbage and pork.

For the cabbage: Gently peel off the leaves of the cabbage. Try to get as many as you can; this is easily done by cutting them at the core. Blanch them in a large pot of salted boiling water for about three minutes until pliable. Drain and set aside.

For the pork filling: In a large frying pan, heat two tablespoons of olive oil, sauté the rosemary and the remaining garlic until it releases its aroma; add the pork until fully cooked. Transfer to a food processor and coarsely chop.

Using the same pan, heat up a tablespoon of olive oil and sauté the onions and celery. When translucent, add the pork and combine. Add some more stock to reach a moist consistency, but be careful to not add too much or it will become runny. The pork should be moist.

Cook for about 10 minutes, then turn off the heat. Add the Parmesan cheese and nutmeg, season with salt and pepper, and combine.

Assemble the parcels by filling a cabbage leaf with the pork stuffing and serve with the tomato sauce.

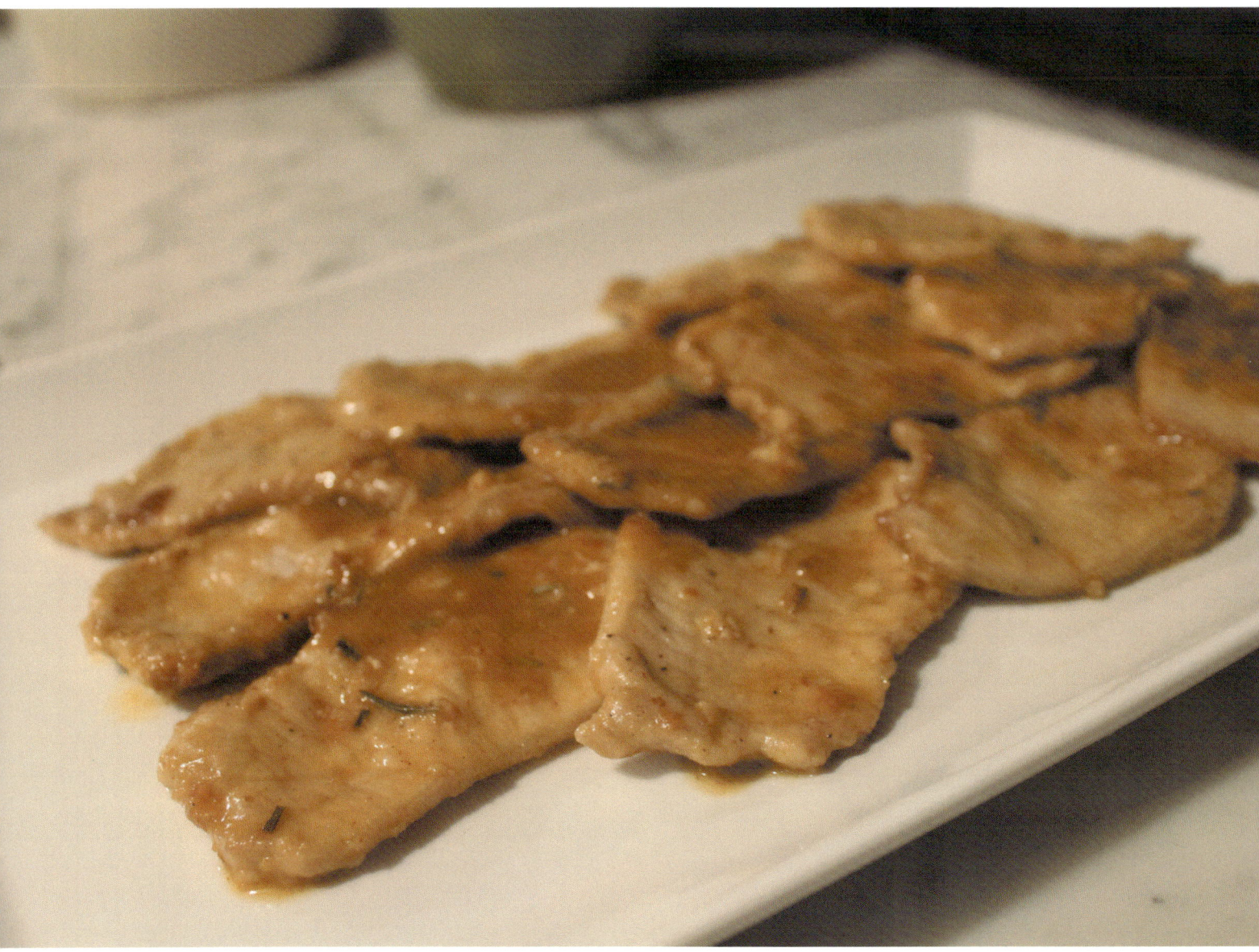

PORK SCALLOPS WITH VERJUICE, ROSEMARY AND GARLIC

Filetto di Maiale con Agresto, Rosmarino e Aglio

Serves 4

Verjuice is an unfermented grape juice typically purchased at a specialty Italian grocery store. If it is not available, you can substitute a good quality white wine such as a Sauvignon Blanc or a Pinot Grigio. Verjuice is not widely known, but in the Middle Ages it was very commonly used for its acidic qualities. We have found when we use verjuice that the overall quality of the dish is elevated.

This recipe pairs this ancient product with rosemary, garlic, and olive oil to create a bright, crisp, tangy sauce for the paper-thin pork scallops.

Ingredients

¼ cup all-purpose flour, to dust the pork scallops

¼ cup olive oil

1 pound of pork loin, cut into very thin slices, approximately one-quarter-inch each

2 teaspoons minced fresh rosemary (or 1 teaspoon dried)

5 cloves of garlic, thinly sliced

¾ cup of verjuice (or white wine if verjuice not available)

Salt and pepper to taste

Season the flour with salt and pepper and lightly cover the pork scallops. Heat the oil in a large skillet over medium-high temperature. Add the pork scallops, taking care not to overcrowd the pan, and sauté about three minutes or until browned. Turn, add rosemary, and cook two to three minutes longer, or until browned on the other side and cooked through. Be careful not to overcook. You will have to do this in two or three batches.

Transfer pork to a platter. To make the sauce, pour the sliced garlic into skillet, cook until it releases its aroma, and do not let it brown.

Add the verjuice and white wine, and begin scraping up any browned bits clinging to the pan, until reduced by about half. Add the pork back to the pan, and cook for about four minutes until the sauce has thickened.

Season with salt and pepper, if needed.

Remove from heat and serve.

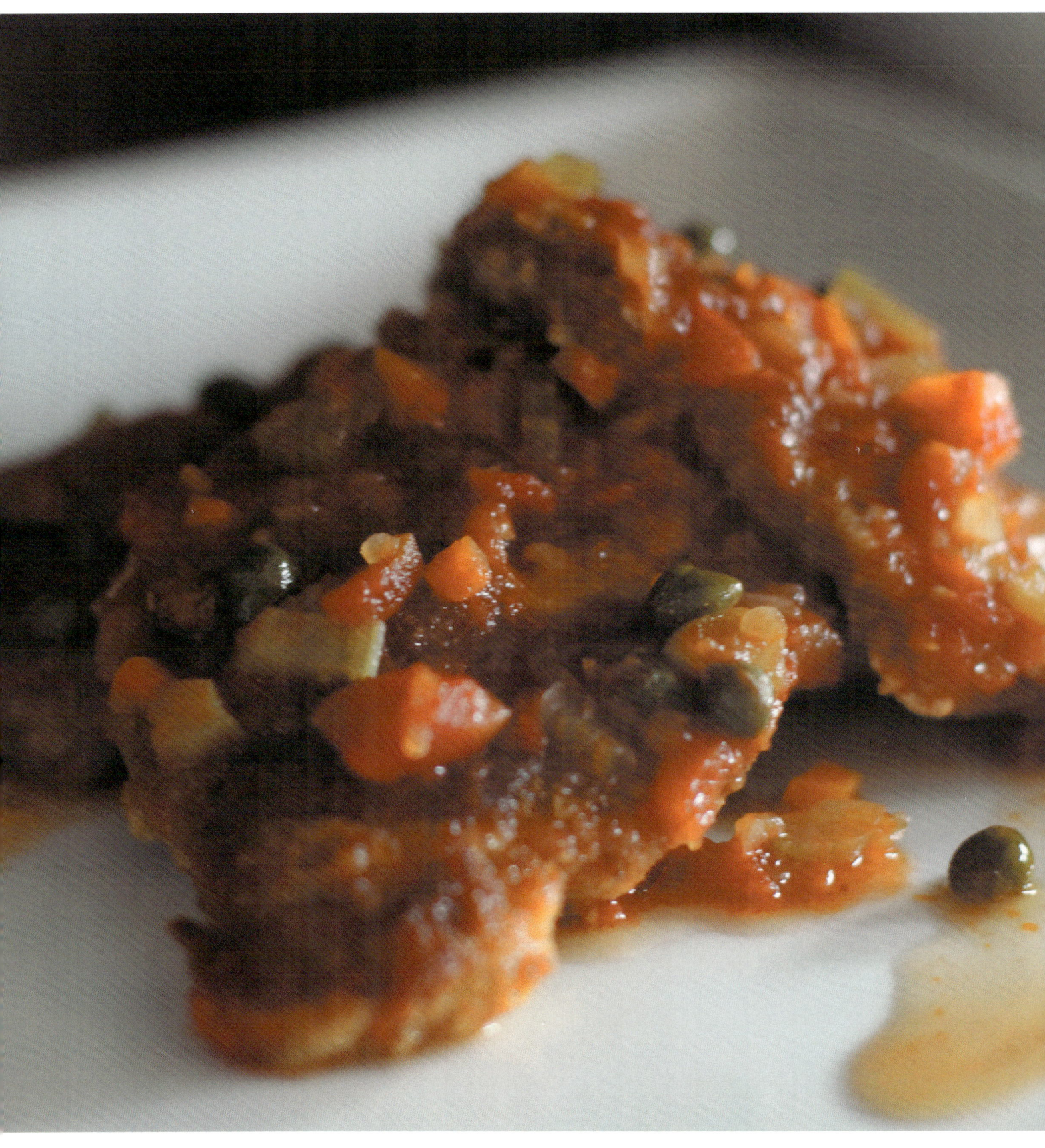

PORK SCALLOPS WITH TOMATO AND CAPER SAUCE, LUCCA STYLE

Filetto di Maiale con Salsa di Pomodoro e Caperi

Serves 4

Popular in the Lucca region, capers are the immature flower buds of the caper bush, which grows in the Mediterranean. We find that capers can be used with many different ingredients to create delicious flavor combinations. Lean pork scallops, instead of the commonly used veal, creates a more affordable and less controversial dinner. We also omit breading and frying the meat; the result is a light and bright dish.

Ingredients

Sea salt and freshly ground pepper to taste

Extra virgin olive oil

1 pound of pork loin sliced half an inch thin

1 medium-size onion, finely chopped

1 cup celery, finely chopped

2 medium-size carrots, finely chopped

1 teaspoon of fresh rosemary, minced

2 cups Italian chopped tomatoes

¼ cup capers, drained and rinsed

1 cup of water

Season the slices of pork with some salt and pepper.

In a large frying pan, heat 4–5 tablespoons of olive oil at medium high heat and cook the pork scallops for about 3–4 minutes on each side. This may require the frying to be done in batches, so replenish the olive oil if needed. When cooked, place the pork on a plate; cover and set aside.

In a large pot, heat 3–4 tablespoons of olive oil at medium-high heat; add the onion, celery, carrots, and rosemary, and cook until translucent. Add the tomatoes, capers, and water, and season with salt and pepper. Cook for about 20 minutes. Then add the pork, combine well, and cook for another 15 minutes.

Do not use too much salt as the capers will release some of their salt while cooking.

Remove from heat and serve hot.

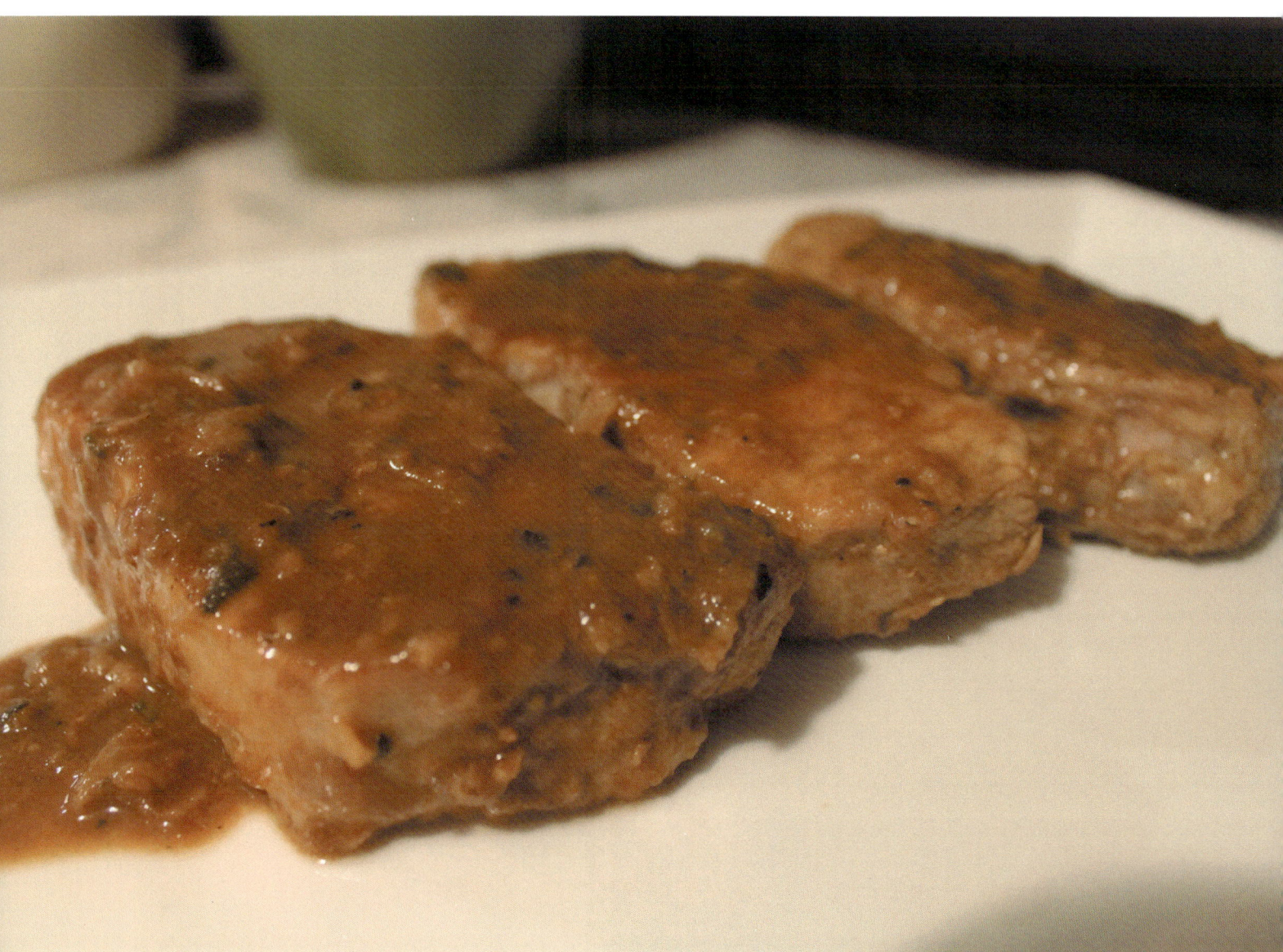

PORK CHOPS WITH BALSAMIC, MUSTARD, AND SAGE

Braciole di Maiale con Aceto Balsamico

Serves 2–4

This is an easy mid-week recipe to make. The fresh sage and mustard with the balsamic vinegar create a tasty sauce without being overwhelming. This dish really is a flavor sensation and a favorite in our household.

Ingredients

4 tablespoons olive oil

All-purpose flour to dust the pork chops (approximately ¼ cup)

Sea salt to taste

1 tablespoon of freshly ground black pepper

4–5 boneless pork chops

2 garlic cloves, minced

4–6 leaves fresh sage, chopped

3 tablespoons Dijon mustard

4 tablespoons balsamic vinegar

¼ cup white wine

½ cup chicken broth

Heat the olive oil over medium heat in a large non-stick skillet. Stir together the flour, salt, and pepper in a pie plate or flat-bottomed bowl. Dredge each pork chop through the flour mixture on all sides and then place the chops in the hot skillet. Let them cook undisturbed for about three minutes.

Flip the chops over; they should be golden brown. Remove them from the pan and keep covered. Keep the same pan at medium heat, and add the garlic, fresh sage and Dijon mustard. Cook for about a minute without browning the garlic. Add the balsamic vinegar and wine until the alcohol has evaporated, then add enough stock to form a sauce. Put the chops back in and cook for an additional three minutes. Flip once more and pour sauce on the pork chops. Remove to a plate and pour any pan juices over the meat. Let rest for five minutes before serving.

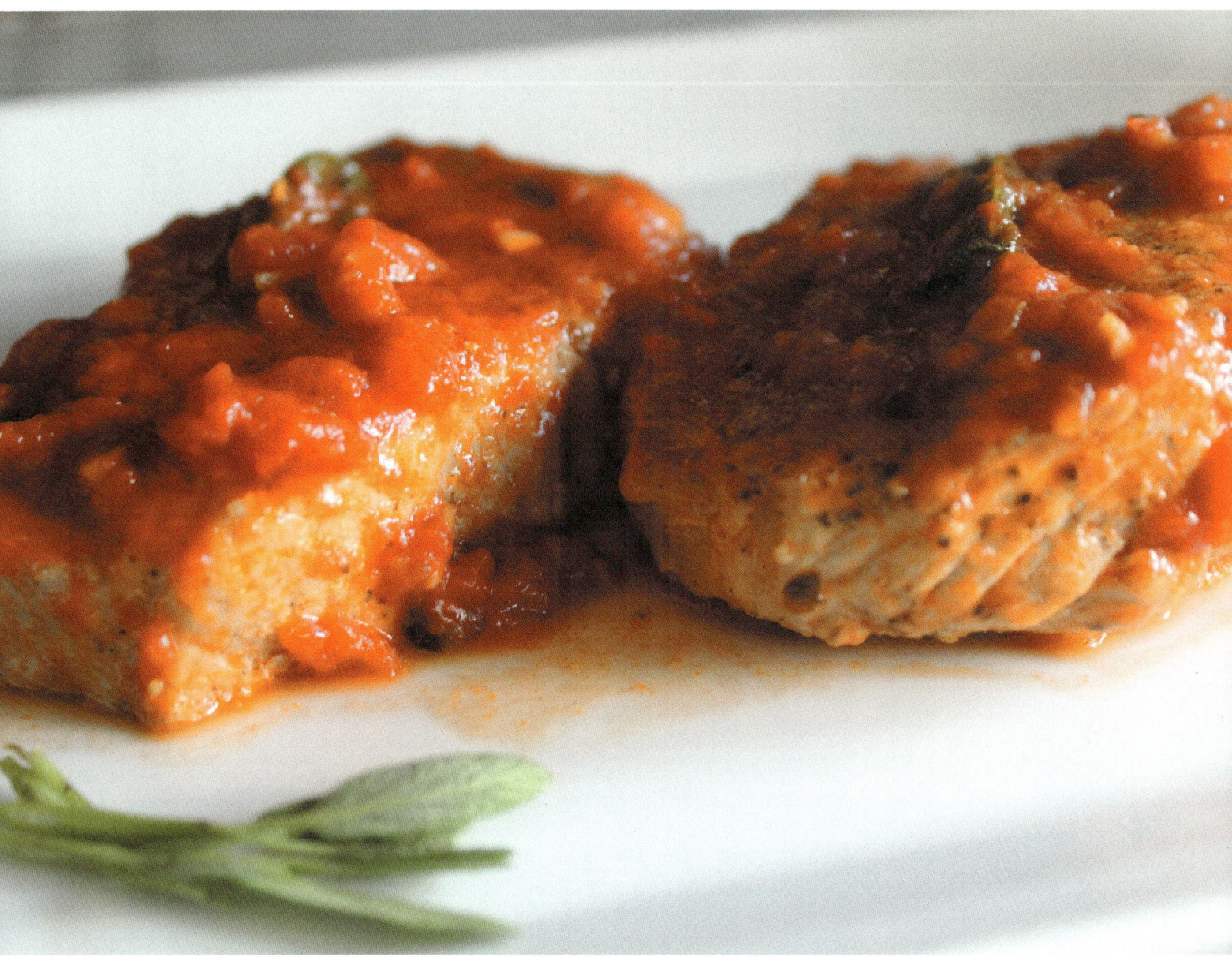

PORK CHOPS WITH TOMATO SAUCE AND FRESH SAGE

Cotolette di Maiale al Pomodoro e Salvia Fresca

Serves 3–4

Fresh sage is assertive, rich, and almost smoky; it enhances the flavor of any meat, particularly pork.

Sage use was not limited to only cooking, according to my teacher in Fiesole. She remembered that during the harsh years of Mussolini's rule, things were so scarce and expensive to obtain that sage leaves were routinely used as improvised toothbrushes.

This is an easy-to-make recipe with just a few ingredients.

Ingredients

4–6 boneless pork chops

1½ tablespoon of freshly ground black pepper

5 tablespoons of extra virgin olive oil

8–10 medium size fresh sage leaves

2 cups chopped Italian tomatoes

2 cloves of garlic finally chopped

Sea salt

1 cup of water

Sprinkle the pork chops with salt and black pepper and set aside.

In a large frying pan, heat (at medium-high) three tablespoons of olive oil. Add four sage leaves and the pork chops without overcrowding the pan; brown both sides of the pork chops for about five or six minutes. Remove from the pan, set aside and discard the oil.

Using the same pan, with the temperature still at medium-high heat, add the remaining two tablespoons of olive oil, remaining sage leaves, and garlic, cooking just long enough for the garlic to release its aroma.

Next, add the tomatoes and water, season with salt, and cook for about 10 minutes.

Add the pork chops to the sauce and cook for another 15–20 minutes. Add water to the sauce if it becomes too dry.

Remove from heat and serve hot.

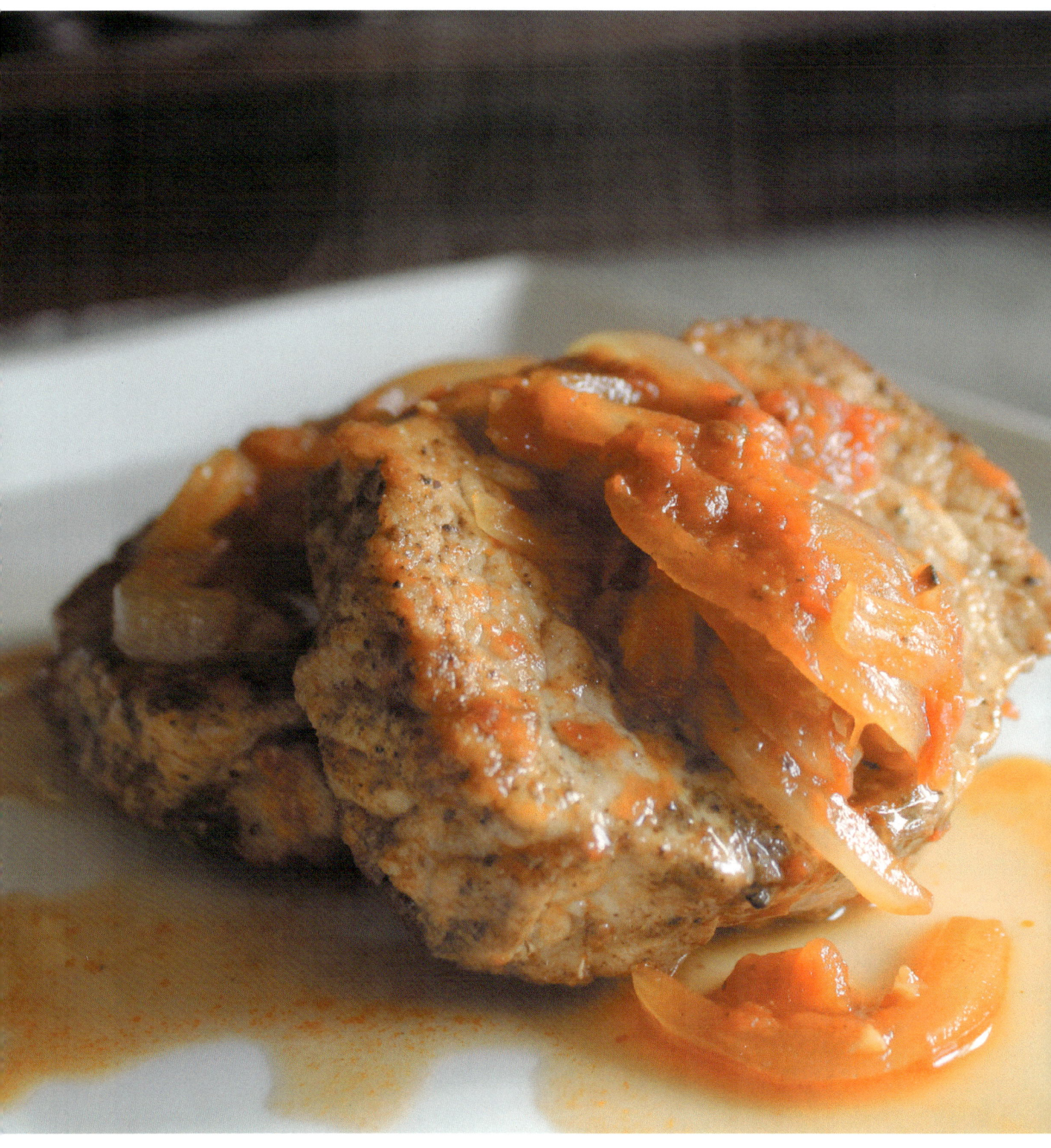

PORK CHOPS WITH ONIONS, TOMATOES AND CUMIN SAUCE

Braciole di Maiale con Salsa de Cipolla, Cumino e Pomodoro

Serves 4

Cumin is more commonly associated with Mexican or Indian cuisines, but it's also been used in Italian kitchens since the the Roman Empire. The large amount of onions add an additional layer of sweetness to the tomatoes.

Ingredients

4 boneless pork chops, extra fat removed

4 tablespoons olive oil

1½ tablespoons ground cumin

1 teaspoon red pepper flakes

1 chopped garlic clove

2 medium-size yellow onions, cut in half-circles

1 cup chopped tomatoes

1 cup chicken stock

Salt to taste

In a frying pan, cook the pork chops in one or two tablespoons of olive oil and brown well on both sides. Take the pork chops out and add a tablespoon of olive oil to the pan, along with the cumin, the red pepper flakes, and the onions; cook at medium heat until onions begin to soften. Add the garlic until it releases its aroma, and do not overcook; add the chopped tomatoes and the chicken stock; mix and season with salt and cook for 10 minutes. Add the pork chops back to the sauce and cook uncovered for another 10 minutes or until fully cooked. Add water or stock to the sauce if it becomes too dry.

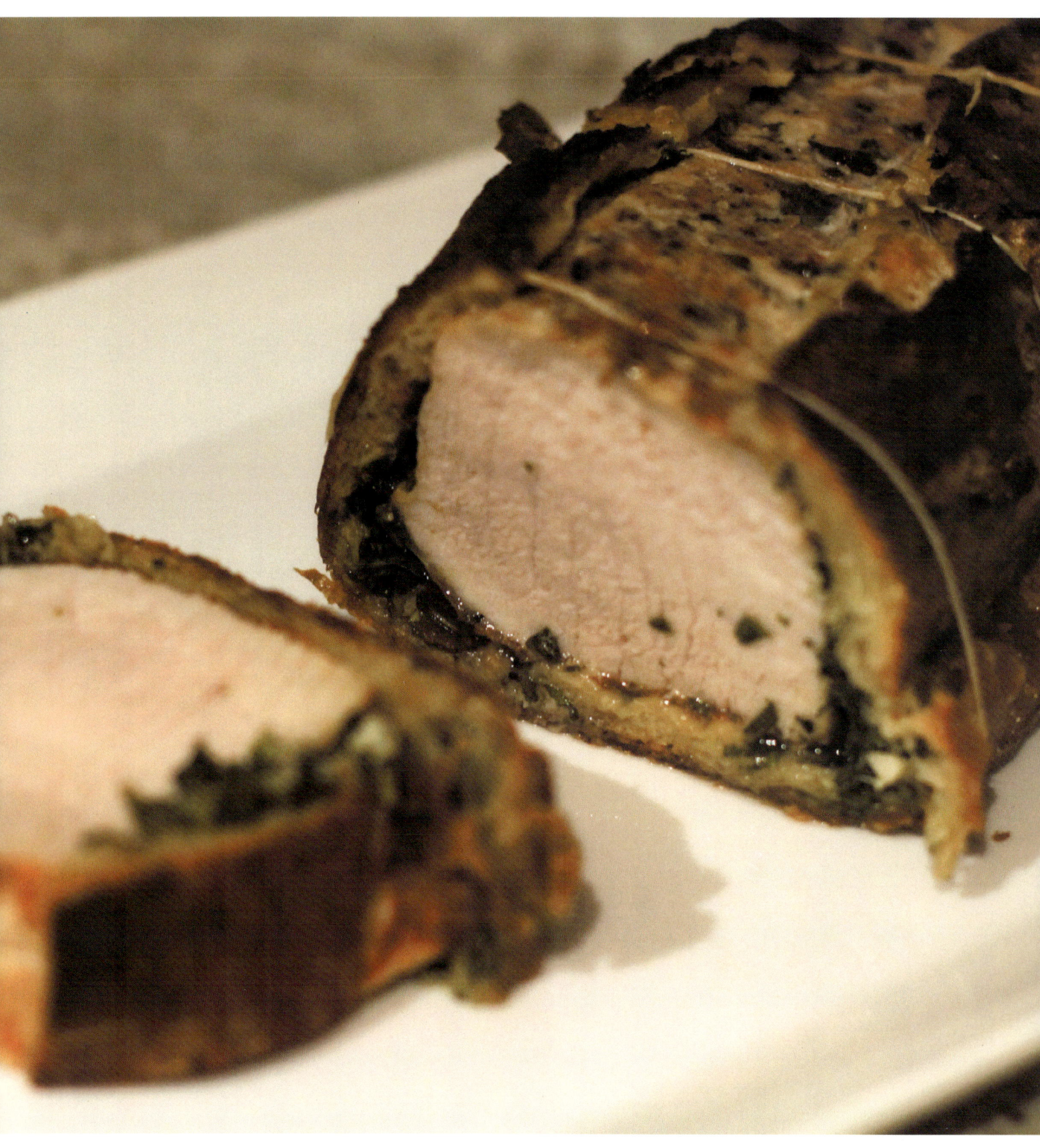

PORK LOIN IN A CRUST OF BREAD

Filetto di Maiale in Crosta di Pane

Serves 4–6

Pork fillet in a crust of bread is a street food that's popular throughout Tuscany, along with *lampredotto*, tripe sandwich. Pork tenderloin is a great cut of meat that is relatively inexpensive, making it even more appealing. Nonna Maria would allow us to stop at the food carts and enjoy this treat while we were out shopping for the evening meal. For this dish, the type of bread plays an important role: it should be crusty with a chewy inside, similar to ciabatta or sourdough. We use the classic Tuscan loaf; while there are those who prefer to cover the fillet with a puff pastry, we prefer the bread, because it better absorbs the flavors of the herbs and pork, and becomes crispy and tasty in the cooking process.

Avoid using soft white Italian-style bread—it will turn to mush, as we discovered through much trial and error.

Ingredients

1 loaf of wide, crusty, baguette-style bread, around fourteen inches long

1 large rosemary sprig, finely chopped to make 1 tablespoon

1 cup chopped fresh basil

1 large clove garlic

4 tablespoons extra virgin olive oil

Sea salt

Black pepper

1 pork tenderloin (3.5–4 pounds) trimmed of any excess fat

Preheat oven to 375°F and set aside some aluminum foil and kitchen twine. Cut the baguette in half across the top, lengthwise, leaving the bottom of the loaf connected. Scoop out some of the soft insides and set aside.

To prepare the herb mixture: Finely chop the rosemary, basil, and garlic, and place in a bowl. Add two to three tablespoons of olive oil and season with sea salt and pepper. Set aside.

To prepare the loin: Heat one tablespoon of olive oil in a large frying pan over medium-high heat. Season the pork tenderloin with salt and ground black pepper. Sear the pork on all sides in the pan and remove after you have a nice golden crust all over the loin.

Spread the herb mixture inside the entire hollow cavity of the bread. Place the pork tenderloin inside the bread and use kitchen twine to secure the bread around the meat. Wrap the baguette tightly in aluminum foil and place on a baking sheet. Bake for about one hour and remove from the oven. Let rest for about 10 minutes and then remove from the foil. If bread is too soggy, you can bake it uncovered for 10–15 more minutes (at the same temperature) until it regains some crunchiness.

Slice and serve hot or at room temperature.

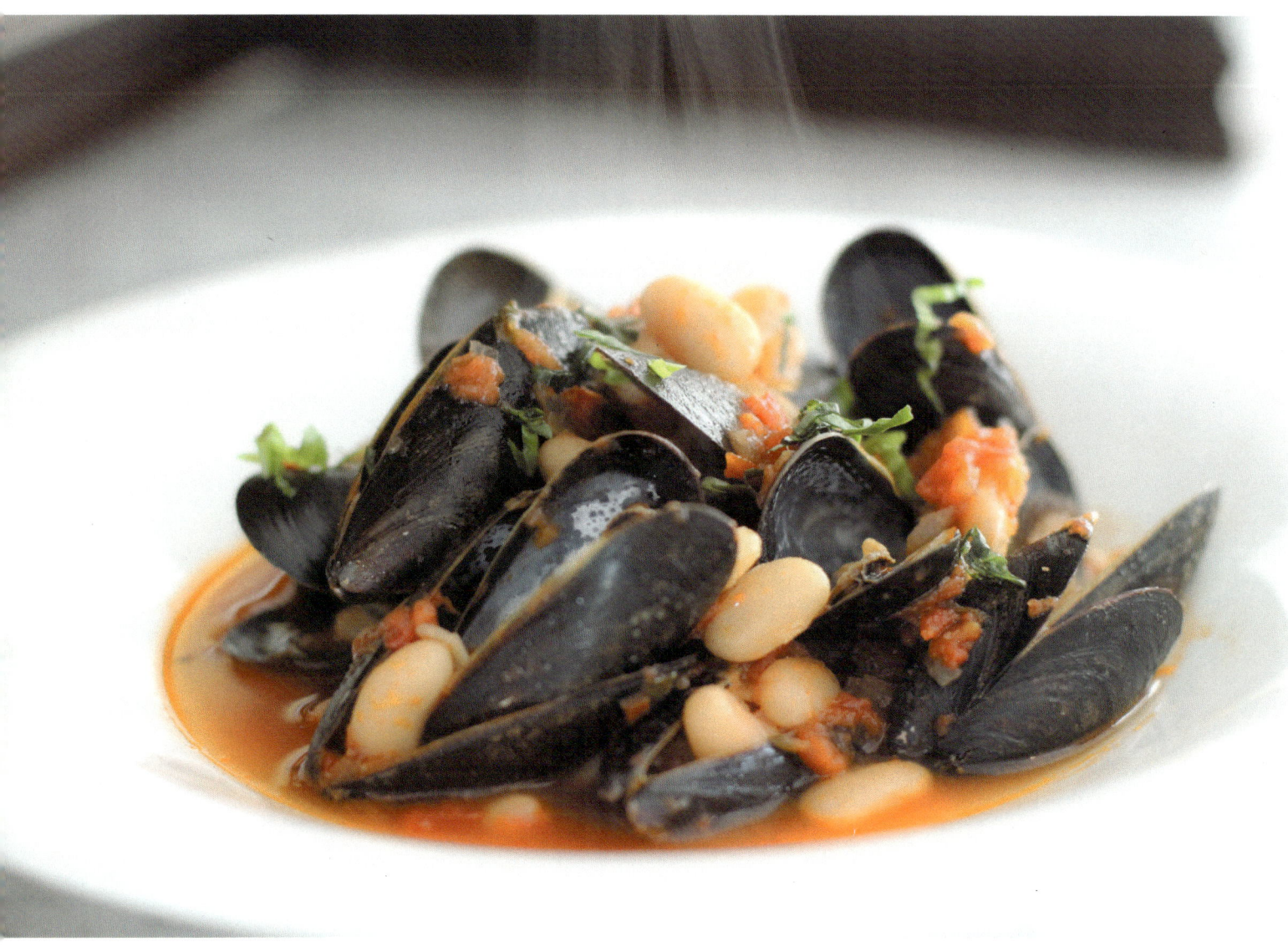

MUSSELS IN TOMATO SAUCE AND CANNELLINI BEANS

Cozze in Salsa di Pomodoro

Serves 4

The mussels are seasoned with just a few basic ingredients. We like to pair this with a nice country bread to sop up the sauce. This is a simple recipe that is light and makes a wonderful summer evening meal.

Ingredients

4 tablespoons extra virgin olive oil

2 cloves garlic, thinly sliced

1½ cups canned Italian chopped tomatoes

1 cup loosely packed fresh basil leaves, chopped

Pepperoncino (red pepper flakes) to taste

Sea salt

1 can (15 ounces) cannellini beans drained and rinsed

2 pounds of fresh mussels, cleaned and with beards removed. Thoroughly clean the mussels under running water, and remove any beards.

Heat four tablespoons of oil in a large pan; add the garlic and brown it slightly (without making it too brown). Add the crushed tomatoes, half of the basil, hot pepper flakes, and salt to taste. Cook for 10 minutes on medium-high heat. Add the cannellini beans and cook for another five minutes.

Add the mussels. Mix them into the sauce, cover the pan, and let the mussels open, discarding the ones that remained closed. Sprinkle with the remaining basil. Put the mussels in individual bowls and serve hot with slices of toasted bread to soak up the delicious juices.

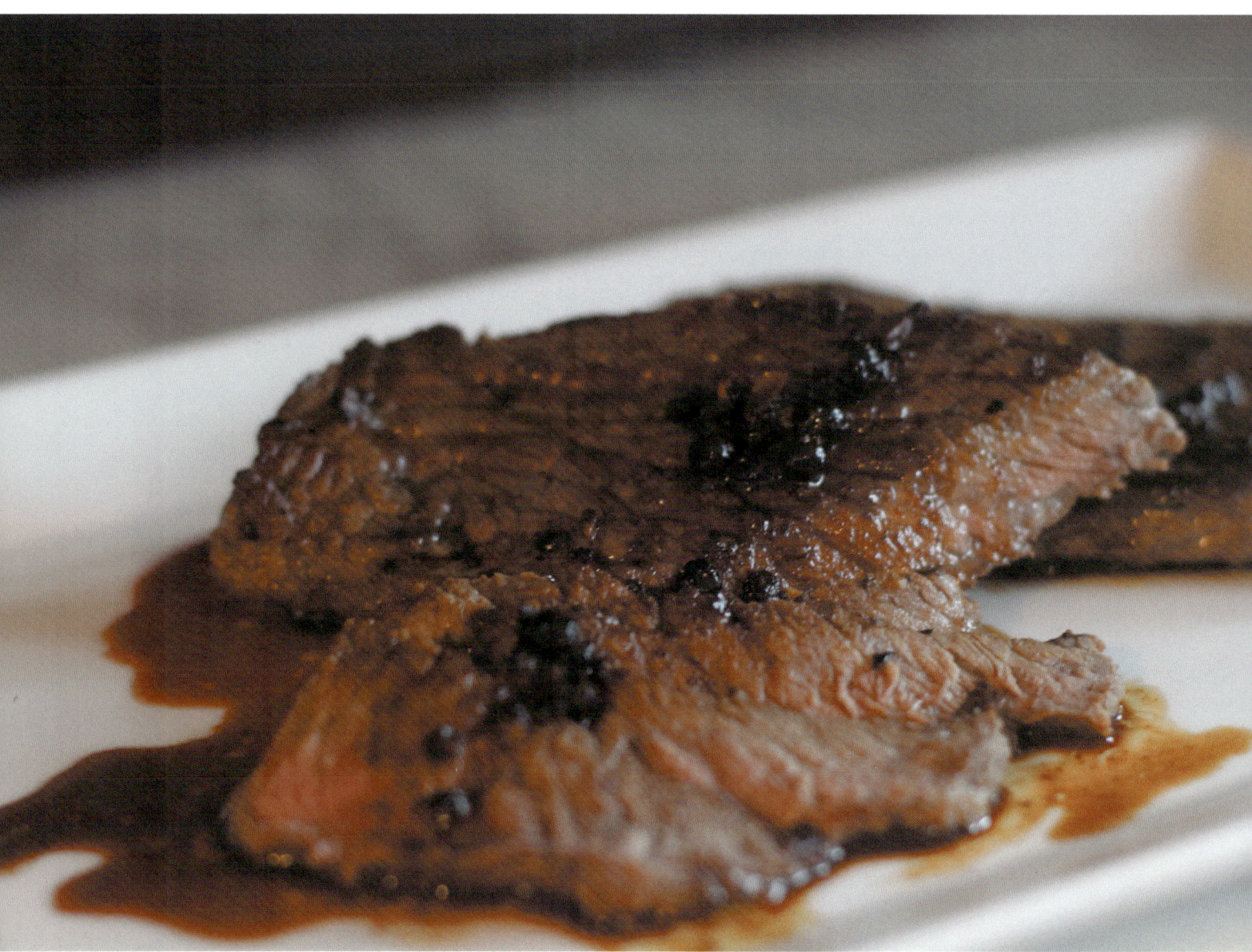

GRILLED STEAKS MARINATED WITH JUNIPER BERRIES AND GARLIC

Bistecca al Ginepro

Serves 4

Juniper berries are traditionally used in cooking wild meats such as the popular *Cinghiale* (Wild Boar) in Tuscany, as well as rabbit, pheasants and other game. This recipe calls for the cut of beef of your choice, scented with juniper berries, rosemary, and garlic. Using this delicious and simple recipe, you can grill, broil, or even sauté the meat.

Ingredients

2 cloves garlic, chopped

1 teaspoon of fresh, finely chopped rosemary

1 tablespoon juniper berries, lightly crushed

Freshly ground black pepper

Sea salt

1½ pounds of your choice of steak, cut into 4 portions

Extra virgin olive oil

Grind together the garlic, the juniper berries, a couple of grinds of black pepper, and a pinch of salt; rub the meat with this mixture. Sprinkle the meat with olive oil and the rosemary, then pop it onto a heated grill or into a pre-heated oven at 420°F in a casserole dish. Roast the meat for 20 minutes if in the oven, or grill it until it reaches your preferred state of doneness.

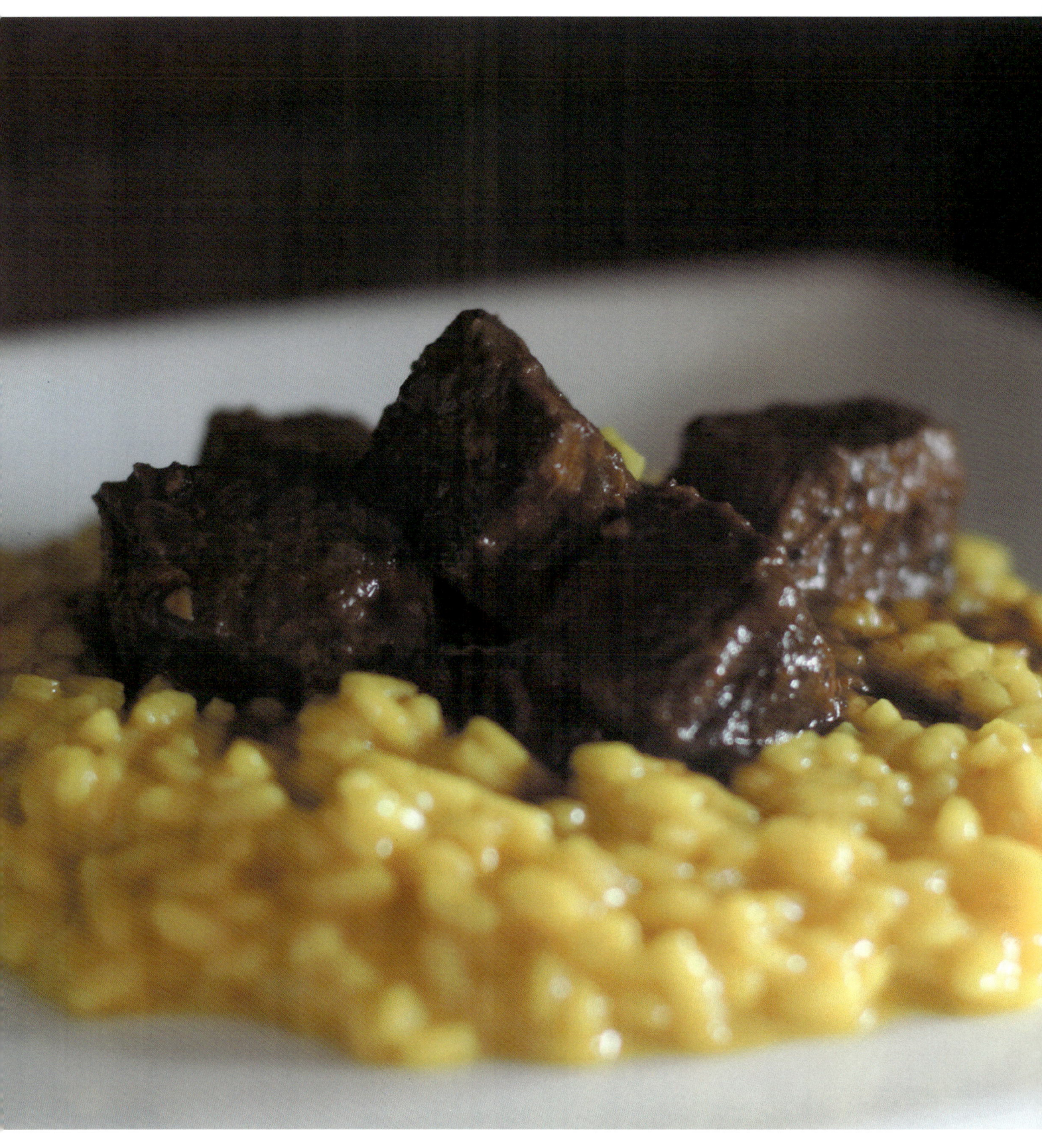

PEPPERY BEEF STEW IMPRUNETA STYLE

Peposo All'Imprunetina

Serves 4

Impruneta, a town just nine miles outside Florence, is known for its production of "cotto" tiles. Peposo All'Imprunetina traces its origins to the same ovens used to manufacture the clay tiles used in Brunelleschi's Duomo in Firenze.

The bold flavors of this recipe are the result of the large amount of black pepper, red wine, and rosemary. We prefer the pre-Columbian version that doesn't include tomatoes—perfect served over saffron risotto (page 65) or polenta.

Ingredients

3 tablespoons of olive oil

2 pounds of beef for stew, cubed and trimmed of all extra fat

1½ tablespoons of freshly ground black pepper

Sea salt

1 large yellow onion, finely chopped

2 tablespoons of fresh rosemary, chopped

3 cups of a good quality red wine; Chianti would be the traditional choice, but a Sangiovese, Cabernet Sauvignon, and Merlot all work well.

2–4 cups of cold water

In a large pot, heat the olive oil at medium high; add the meat, pepper, and salt to taste, and brown for about 20–25 minutes. Add the onions and rosemary and continue cooking until the onion is soft.

Add the wine and two cups of water; bring to a simmer, reduce the heat, and cook covered for 60–90 minutes. Check the tenderness of the meat; if more cooking time is needed, make sure to add enough extra water and cook until meat is tender. Do not let the sauce become too dry.

Serve hot over plain polenta or saffron risotto.

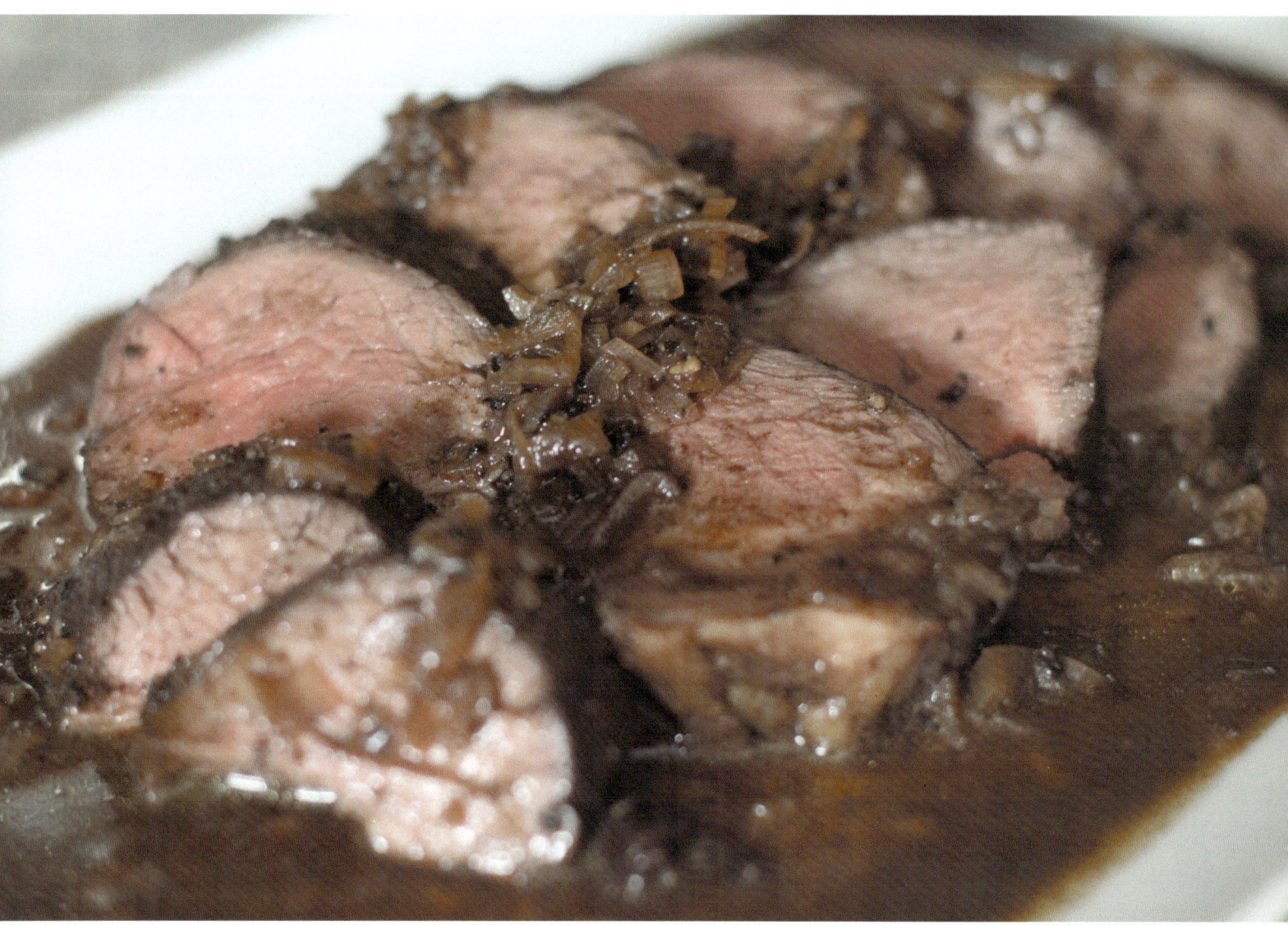

BEEF TENDERLOIN WITH RED WINE AND SHALLOTS

Filetto di Manso al Vino Rosso e Scalogno

Serves 2

A delicious steak fillet that is simple to prepare, flavored with a reduction of red wine, balsamic vinegar, and garlic.

Ingredients

2 fillets of beef

Sea salt and pepper to taste

1 tablespoon of olive oil

2 medium shallots, chopped

4 tablespoons red wine

4 tablespoons of balsamic vinegar

Season the fillet with the salt and pepper from both sides.

Heat the oil in a frying pan and cook the meat for four minutes per side. Using tongs, remove the meat from the pan, keep warm on a plate, and remove the oil from the pan.

Return the pan to the heat and add the shallots. Cook, stirring, for about one minute or until the shallots are thoroughly wilted. Pour the wine and, with a wooden spoon, scrape the bottom of the pan, stirring constantly. Lower the heat and add the balsamic vinegar and continue cooking on low heat until the sauce is reduced to about half.

Return the tenderloin to the pan and let it cook for a few more minutes. Remove from heat and serve with the sauce.

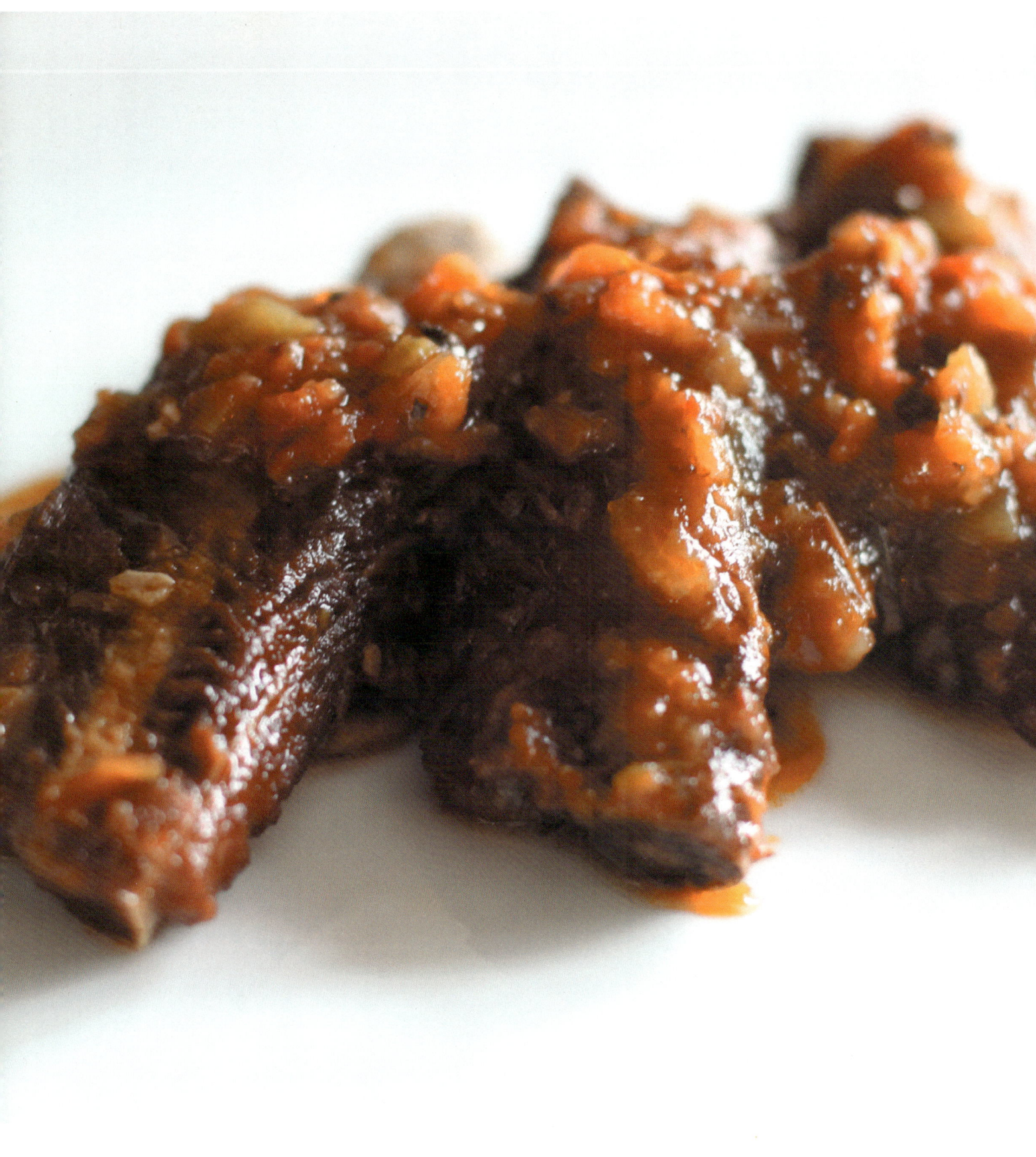

BABY BACK RIBS WITH TOMATOES AND SAGE

Costine di Maiale al Sugo di Pomodoro e Salvia

Serves 4-5

Outside the group of women that ruled the kitchen in my family, a few other women were able to influence me on what to cook and eat: Marcella Hazan was one of those who inspired my fascination with Italian cooking by showing me simple and delicious recipes with very few ingredients.

Ingredients

½ cup chopped celery

½ cup chopped carrots

1 large yellow onion, finely chopped

3 tablespoons olive oil

3 pounds of baby back ribs, divided into single ribs

Sea salt to taste

Black pepper to taste

2 cloves of garlic

1¼ cup red wine

2½ cups chopped Italian plum tomatoes

6-8 large fresh sage leaves

1 cup water or chicken stock (more if necessary)

Chop the celery, carrots, and onion.

In a large sauté pan, which should be large enough to hold all the ribs, heat the olive oil at medium heat and pan roast the ribs until golden brown all over. Reduce or remove the browning oil, add the chopped vegetables, and season with salt and pepper. Continue cooking until translucent. Add garlic and cook briefly until it releases its aroma.

Add the wine and cook until it evaporates; then add the chopped tomatoes and sage as well as the cup of water or chicken stock. Cook covered for 60–90 minutes, at medium-low heat. Make sure the sauce doesn't go dry; keep adding more water if needed.

After 60–90 minutes, the ribs should be tender and the meat should come easily off the bone. Remove from heat and serve hot with a good Tuscan bread to soak up all the juices.

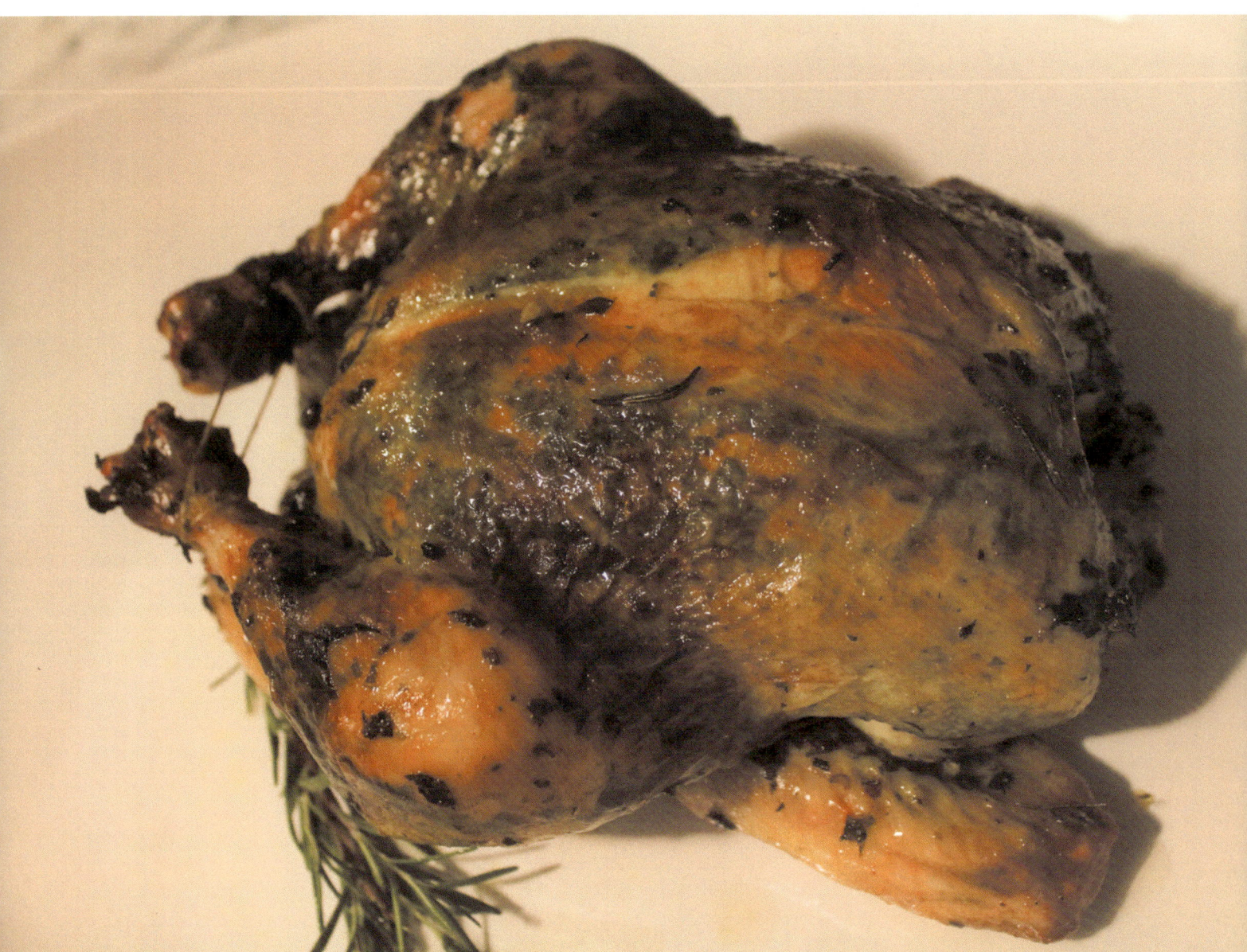

ROASTED CHICKEN WITH FRESH HERBS

Pollo Arrosto Alle Erbe Aromatiche

Serves 4

Try our version of this easy, tasty and time-less classic. The chicken is roasted whole with a blend of aromatic herbs under the skin. This is a more flavorful, fresh, and healthy alternative to the bland supermarket rotis-serie chicken.

Ingredients

1 whole chicken, 3–4 pounds

1½ teaspoons salt plus extra 1 teaspoon to sprinkle the outside of the chicken.

1 tablespoon fresh rosemary, finely chopped

3 fresh sage leaves, finely chopped

1 small bunch fresh basil, chopped (about 1 cup)

2 cloves garlic

4 tablespoons olive oil

Pre-heat oven to 420°F.

Clean the chicken and remove the giblets and any extra fat. Finely chop all the herbs and garlic together. Add the salt, place together inside a small bowl, and add three tablespoons of olive oil. Mix everything well and set aside

Sprinkle chicken with the remaining 1 tablespoon of olive oil and 1 teaspoon of salt.

Insert your fingers between the skin and meat, starting at the neck area and going down to the thighs and legs.

Spread your herb mixture underneath the skin of the chicken. With twine, tie the legs together and fold the wings under the body of the chicken.

Place the chicken in a baking dish, cover with aluminum foil, and roast for one hour.

After one hour, uncover the chicken, baste the chicken with the juices several times, and continue cooking until it is golden and crispy.

Serve the chicken hot.

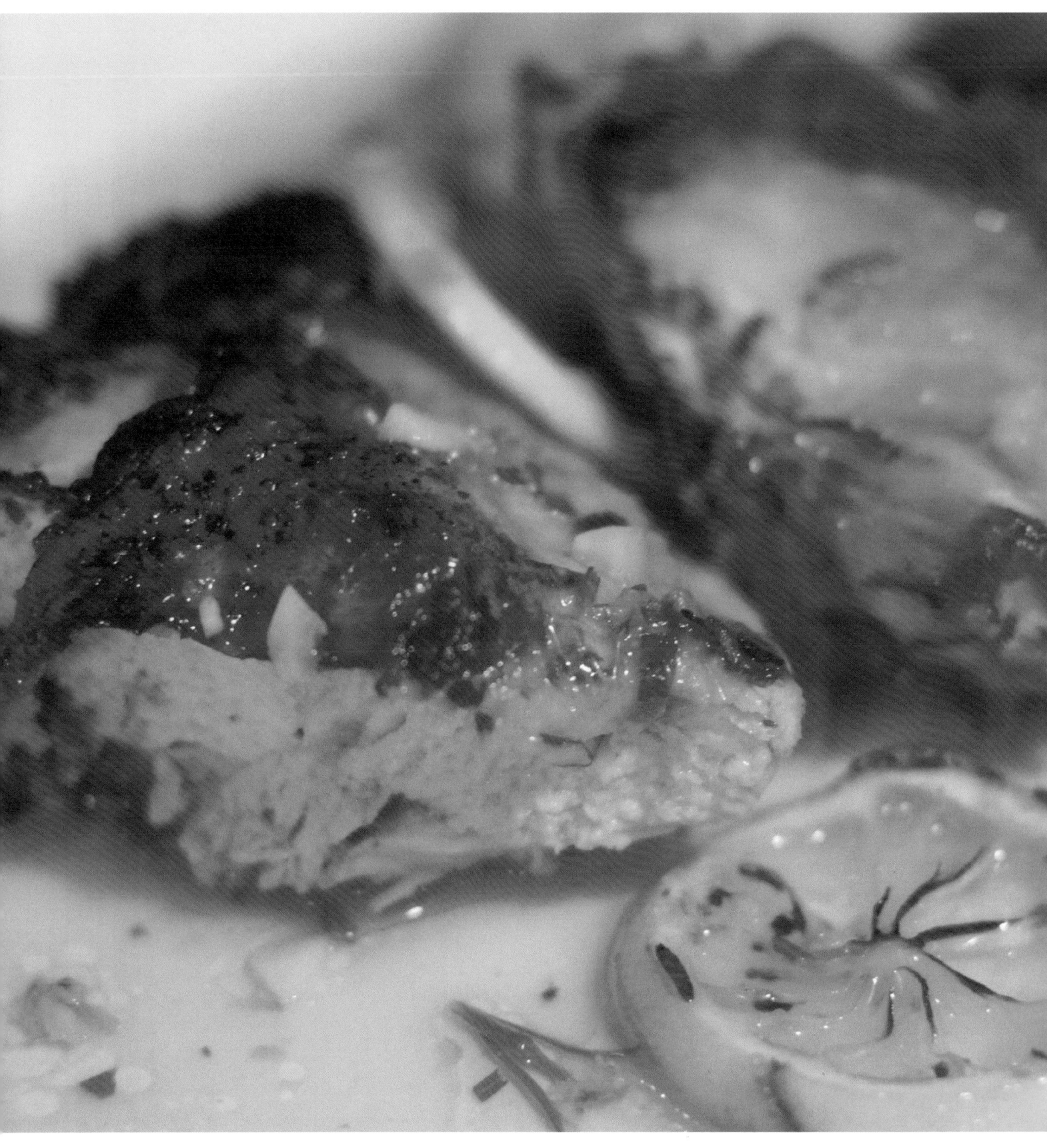

TUSCAN CHICKEN WITH LEMON AND ROSEMARY

Pollo Alla Toscana con Limone e Rosmarino

Serves 4

Easy and tasty roast chicken—and the combination of lemon, rosemary and garlic in this chicken imparts a distinctive flavor. A signature dish in our home, we usually prepare and serve this in a beautiful antique Italian roasting pan we found in a flea market in New Haven, CT.

Ingredients

1 (3½ pound) chicken, cut in half

Sea salt

¼ cup extra virgin olive oil plus 2 tablespoons

⅓ cup freshly squeezed lemon juice

1 tablespoon red wine vinegar

4 garlic cloves, minced

2 fresh rosemary springs, finely chopped

Red pepper flakes

1 lemon cut into thin slices

Make the sauce by combining the lemon juice, olive oil, vinegar, red pepper flakes, garlic, and rosemary; season with salt. Cover and refrigerate until ready to use.

Turn on oven broiler to high and move the oven grill down to a roasting position.

Use the two remaining tablespoons of olive oil to coat the chicken. In a baking pan, turn the chicken breast side down and place in the oven under the broiler. Keep an eye on the oven, and when the chicken is just starting to brown, turn the chicken over (breast side up) and let the skin brown a little. Remove from the broiler and turn the oven temperature down to 375°F.

Cut up the chicken into smaller pieces (up to eight). Pour the lemon and rosemary sauce and lemon slices over the chicken; roast for about 25–30 minutes, basting the sauce over the chicken continuously.

When the chicken is fully cooked, remove from the oven and serve.

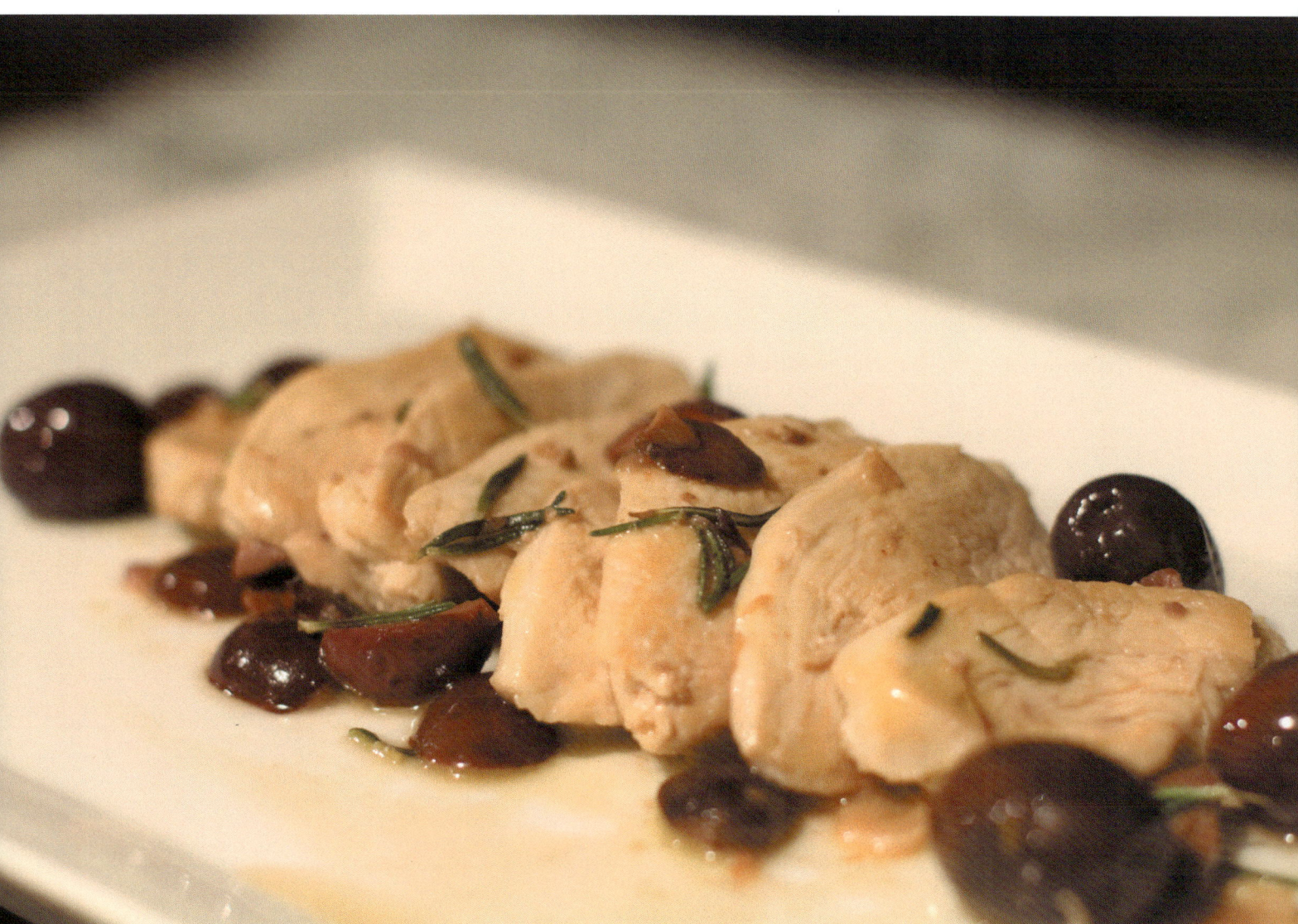

CHICKEN BREAST WITH BLACK OLIVES AND ROSEMARY

Petti di Pollo con Olive alla Toscana

Serves 4-5

Olives were a staple of my existence while growing up. During harvest time, my grandmother would throw olive pits into the oven to turn them to ash, and would mix it with extra virgin olive oil and other ingredients to make her own soap, with which she would wash her perfectly groomed, pitch-black hair. She always looked imposing and elegant, even during the most unbearable days of summer when we would escape the city for the mountains up north.

Rosemary was another ubiquitous ingredient. It was not just used for its flavor but also for its medicinal benefits. Rosemary was traditionally used to alleviate muscle pain, improve memory, and boost the immune system. In Spain and Italy it has been considered a safeguard from witches and evil.

This quick and easy recipe reminds me of those days.

Ingredients

3 tablespoons of extra virgin olive oil

1 cup of black olives marinated in olive oil; do not use canned or brined in water

1 medium-size onion, finely chopped

4 halves of boneless and skinless chicken breast

1 small spring of fresh rosemary, chopped

2 cloves of garlic, minced

1 cup of white wine

Sea salt

Black pepper

Cut the boneless/skinless chicken breast into one-inch slices.

In a large sauté pan, heat the olive oil at medium heat; add half of the olives and all of the onion, cooking until the onion is soft; add the chicken, rosemary, and the garlic.

Cook long enough for the chicken to cook through, approximately 15 minutes; by now, a thick sauce should be forming. Add the wine and combine well, cooking until the alcohol has evaporated.

Season with salt and pepper and add the remaining olives. Cook for another eight to ten minutes.

Remove from heat and serve hot.

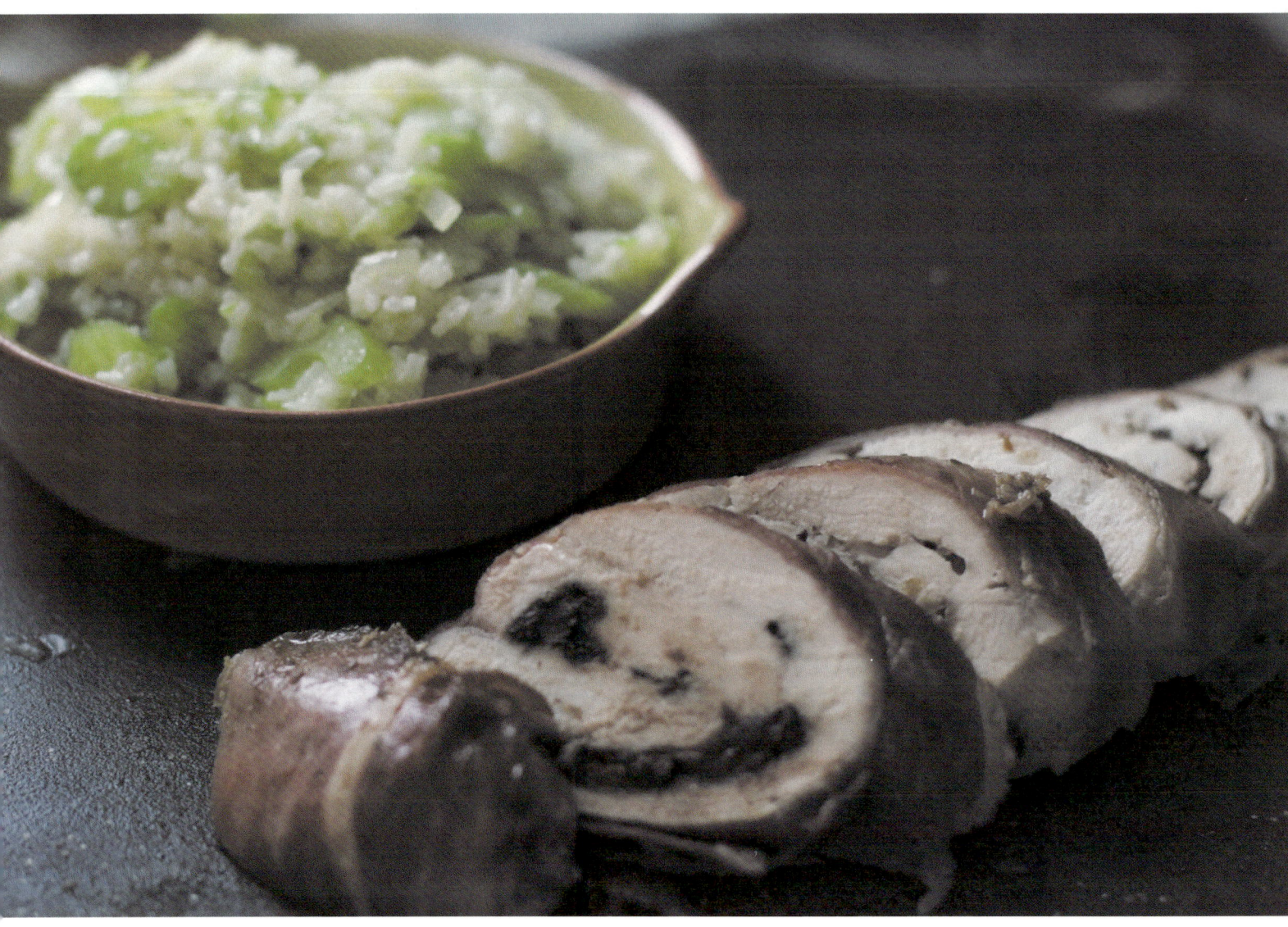

CHICKEN BREAST STUFFED WITH BLACK OLIVES AND WRAPPED IN PROSCIUTTO

Cotoletta di Pollo Con Olive e Prosciutto

Serves 2

This recipe was created by accident by using the few ingredients we had available during a snowstorm that prevented us from reaching the supermarket.

This dish may sound complicated, but is relatively easy to make. Leftover olives, rosemary, and cheese become the filling. The chicken breast, wrapped in prosciutto, remains moist and flavorful.

Ingredients

1 cup of black olives, marinated in olive oil, chopped

Olive oil

1 teaspoon of fresh rosemary, chopped

4 halves of boneless chicken breast

1 cup of cheese, grated (montasio is our favorite, but an aged asiago would work.)

2 packs of prosciutto

1 cup of white wine

Pre-heat oven to 375°F.

In a bowl, mix the olives and rosemary.

To form pockets in each chicken breast, cut a three-inch-long slit in the thick side of each breast, cutting into breast about two inches and to within half an inch of the opposite side, making sure not to cut all the way through.

Fill the pockets with the olive mix and some cheese; wrap the breast in prosciutto and tie with three pieces of kitchen twine. The chicken doesn't need to be seasoned with salt, as there is enough salt in the olives and prosciutto.

Place on a baking dish and bake for about 35–40 minutes or until completely done. Remove from the pan and cut into medallions.

Deglaze the pan to make a sauce with white wine; reduce until the alcohol from the wine has evaporated, and drizzle on top of the chicken.

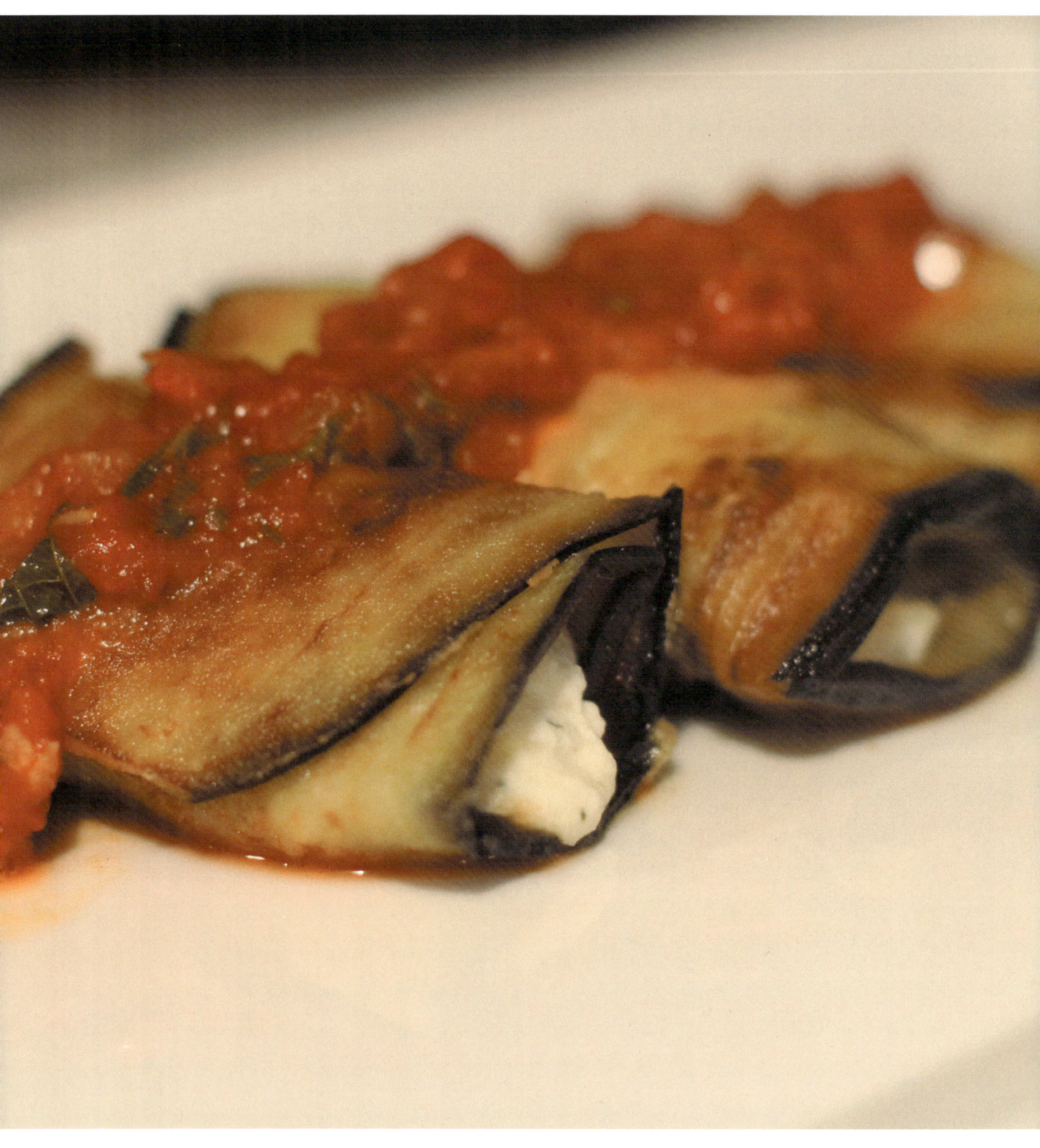

EGGPLANT ROLLS WITH RICOTTA IN A TOMATO, BASIL, AND MINT SAUCE

Involtino de Melanzana in Salsa di Pomodoro con Basilico e Menta

Serves 4

In America, mint is not usually added to a tomato sauce, but in Italy I learned to add it to both tomato sauce and pesto. This is a light and delicious dish, with the smoky flavor of the eggplant enhanced by fresh mint.

Ingredients for the sauce

4 tablespoons olive oil

1 small yellow onion, chopped

1 garlic clove, chopped

2 cups chopped tomatoes, peeled and seeded

½ cup fresh basil, finely chopped

½ cup fresh mint, no stems finely chopped

1 cup water

Salt and pepper to taste

Ingredients for the eggplant and filling

¼ cup olive oil

1¼ pound eggplant, cut in quarter-inch lengthwise slices

1 cup fresh ricotta cheese

¼ cup Parmesan cheese

Zest of 1 lemon

2 tablespoons fresh basil, chopped

All-purpose flour for dusting

For the sauce:

Heat a large saucepan at medium heat with four tablespoons of olive oil; add the chopped onions until translucent. Add the garlic, but do not let it brown. Add the tomatoes and bring to a boil. Then, add the basil, mint, and water, and simmer uncovered for about 10 minutes. Season with salt and pepper to taste.

For the eggplant:

Dust the eggplant slices with flour and set aside.

Heat a large, non-stick skillet over medium heat. Add one-quarter cup of olive oil to cook the eggplant slices in a single layer in batches until light brown and pliable (one minute per side) and place on a tray.

For the filling:

In a large bowl, combine the ricotta, Parmesan cheese, lemon zest, basil, and two tablespoons of olive oil; season with salt and pepper.

Place one tablespoon of the cheese mixture on each eggplant slice and roll, pressing gently to obtain a slightly flat shape.

Pour sauce on a plate and place rolls on top of it, and garnish with more sauce on top.

Serve immediately.

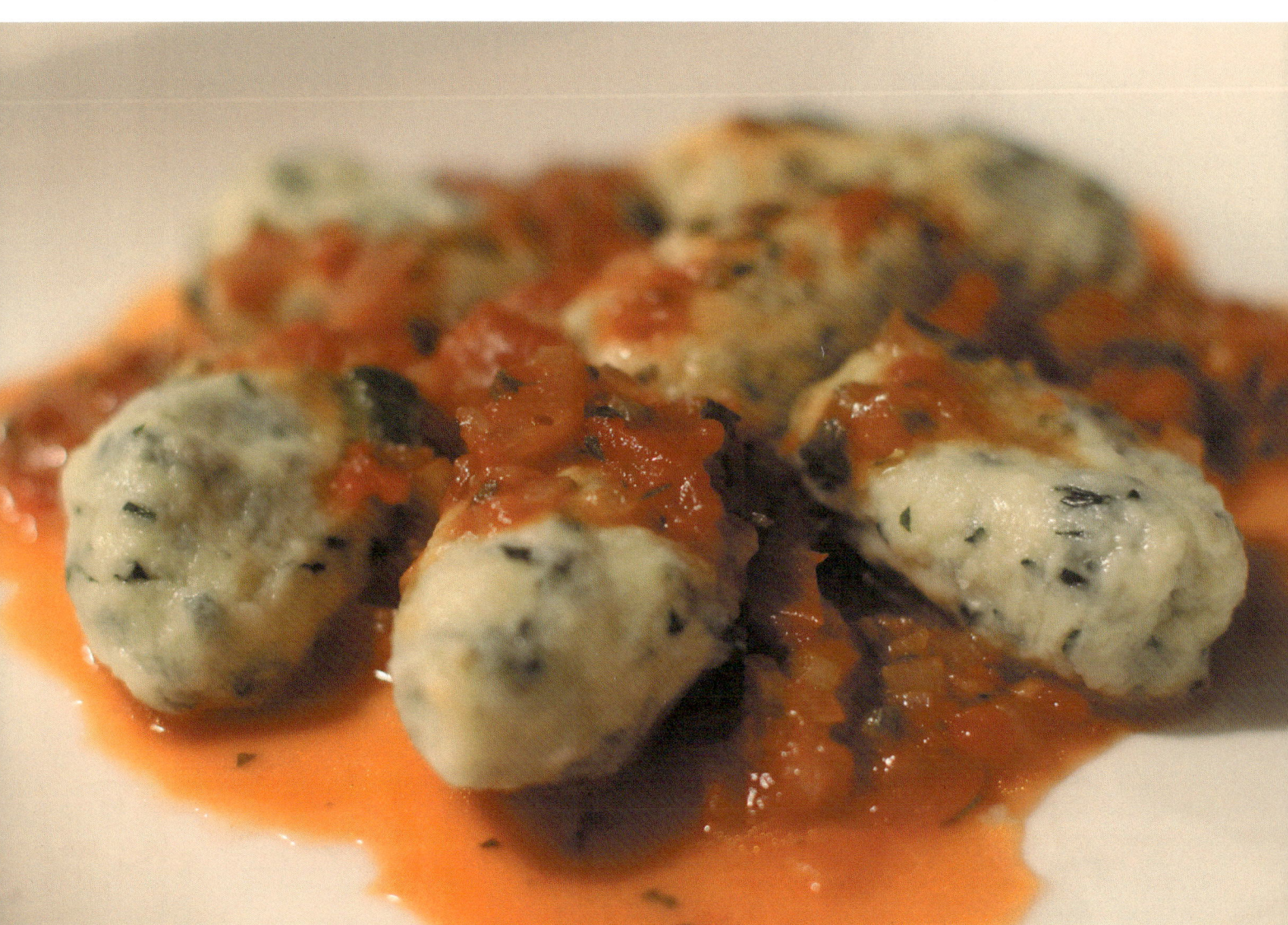

NAKED RAVIOLI WITH BASIL SCENTED TOMATO SAUCE

Gnudi o Malfatti con Salsa di Pomodoro al Basilico

Serves 4–6

Gnudi or naked ravioli may not look very beautiful, but their taste is rich and satisfying. They are also known as *malfatti* ("badly made") in Italian because of their uneven shape. This is one of the few pasta dishes found throughout Tuscany, but the main ingredient is ricotta rather than wheat flour.

Gnudi can be served with a simple basil tomato sauce or butter with fresh sage. Both recipes can be found here.

Ingredients

1 pound spinach, stalks removed and rinsed

2 eggs, lightly beaten

1 cup ricotta cheese

¾ cup all-purpose flour, plus extra for dusting (We use Italian "oo" flour, but if you cannot find this, you may use all-purpose flour.)

1 cup grated Parmesan cheese, plus extra for serving

¼ teaspoon grated nutmeg

Salt and pepper

Quick Tomato Sauce with Fresh Basil (see recipe on page 7)

Cook the spinach in lightly salted boiling water for five minutes. It is very important to drain the spinach very well; when it cools down, use your hands to squeeze out any excess liquid. Chop spinach finely and place into a bowl with the eggs, ricotta, flour, Parmesan, nutmeg and a pinch of salt. Mix well.

Sprinkle your work surface or a large plate with some flour and use a teaspoon to begin creating little round balls. Prepare another pot of salted water and bring to a boil; water should remain at a gentle boil, otherwise your gnudi will disintegrate. Lightly drop the gnudi into the pot.

When the gnudi are ready, which should be in four minutes more or less, they will pop to the surface. Begin collecting and draining them with a skimmer.

Serve with your choice of sauce—we prefer the Quick Tomato Sauce with Fresh Basil— and garnish with more Parmesan cheese. Alternatively, you could try it with a butter and sage sauce, described in the Nude Ravioli recipe on page 125.

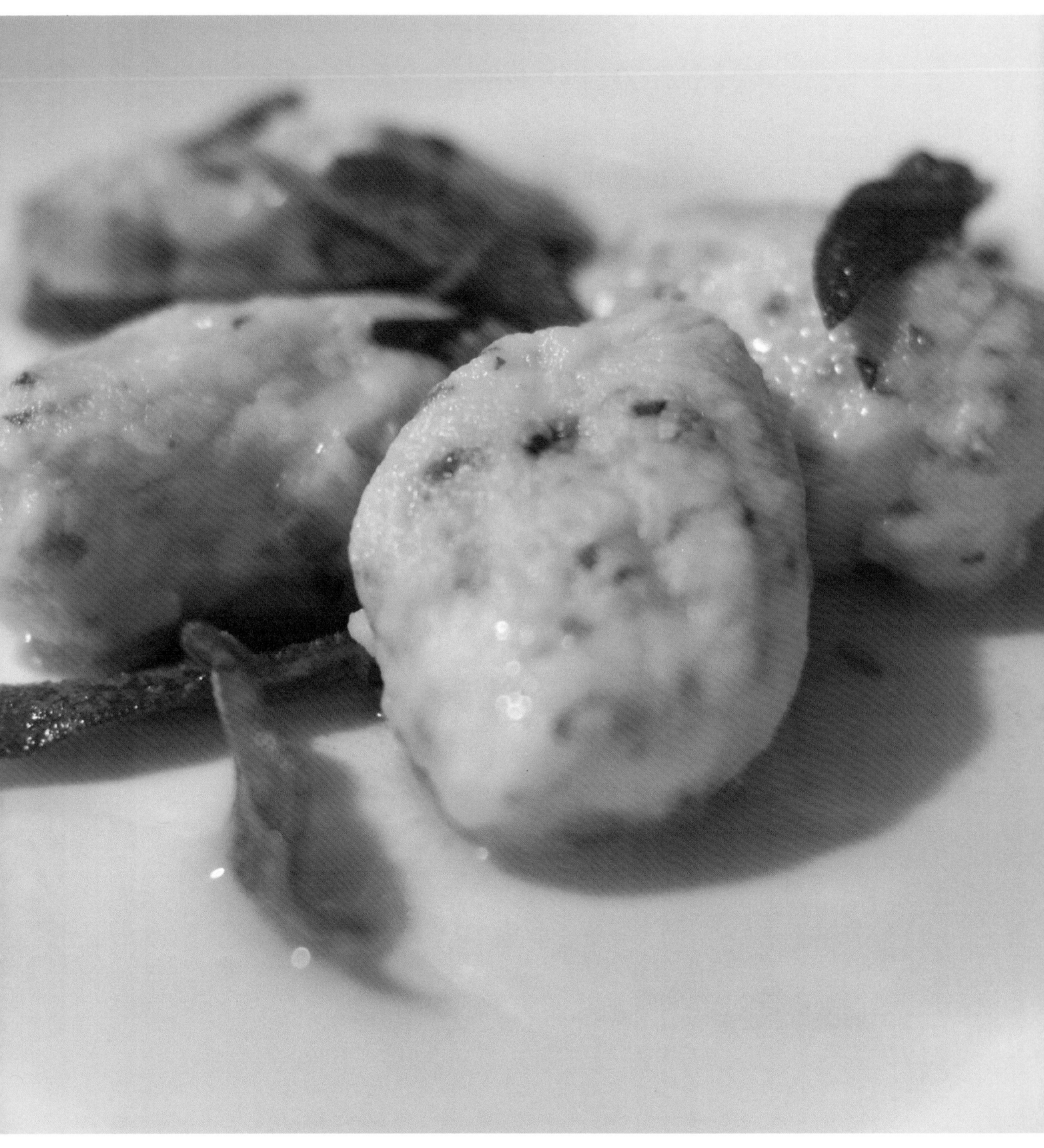

NUDE RAVIOLI
Gnudi

Serves 4

A simple sauce made with butter and sage make this dish a perfect example of the uncomplicated approach of Italian cooking.

Ingredients

One (16 ounces) bag of fresh spinach

1 cup ricotta cheese

1 cup grated Parmesan cheese

2 eggs, lightly beaten

¾ cup all-purpose flour, plus more for dusting the dumplings (We use Italian "00" flour, but if you cannot find this, you may use all-purpose flour.)

½ teaspoon of nutmeg

Sea salt and freshly ground pepper

3 tablespoons olive oil

12 fresh sage leaves

3 tablespoons butter

For the gnudi:

Rinse the spinach and cook in a pan covered for about five minutes; no oil or salt is needed. Drain the spinach as much as you can, and once it's cooled, chop it.

In a large bowl, mix the ricotta, Parmesan, beaten eggs, flour and nutmeg. Season with salt and pepper.

Bring a large pot of salted water to a boil.

We found the easiest way to form the dumplings is to use a teaspoon and dust them with flour. Cook them in batches, making sure not to crowd the pot. They are ready in three to four minutes, and will float when ready.

Remove from the boiling water and drain them on paper towels; keep them warm.

For the sauce:

In a saucepan, heat olive oil at medium and add the sage leaves; cook until the leaves turn golden brown and add the butter to finish the sauce.

Plate the dumplings and drizzle the sauce over. Serve immediately.

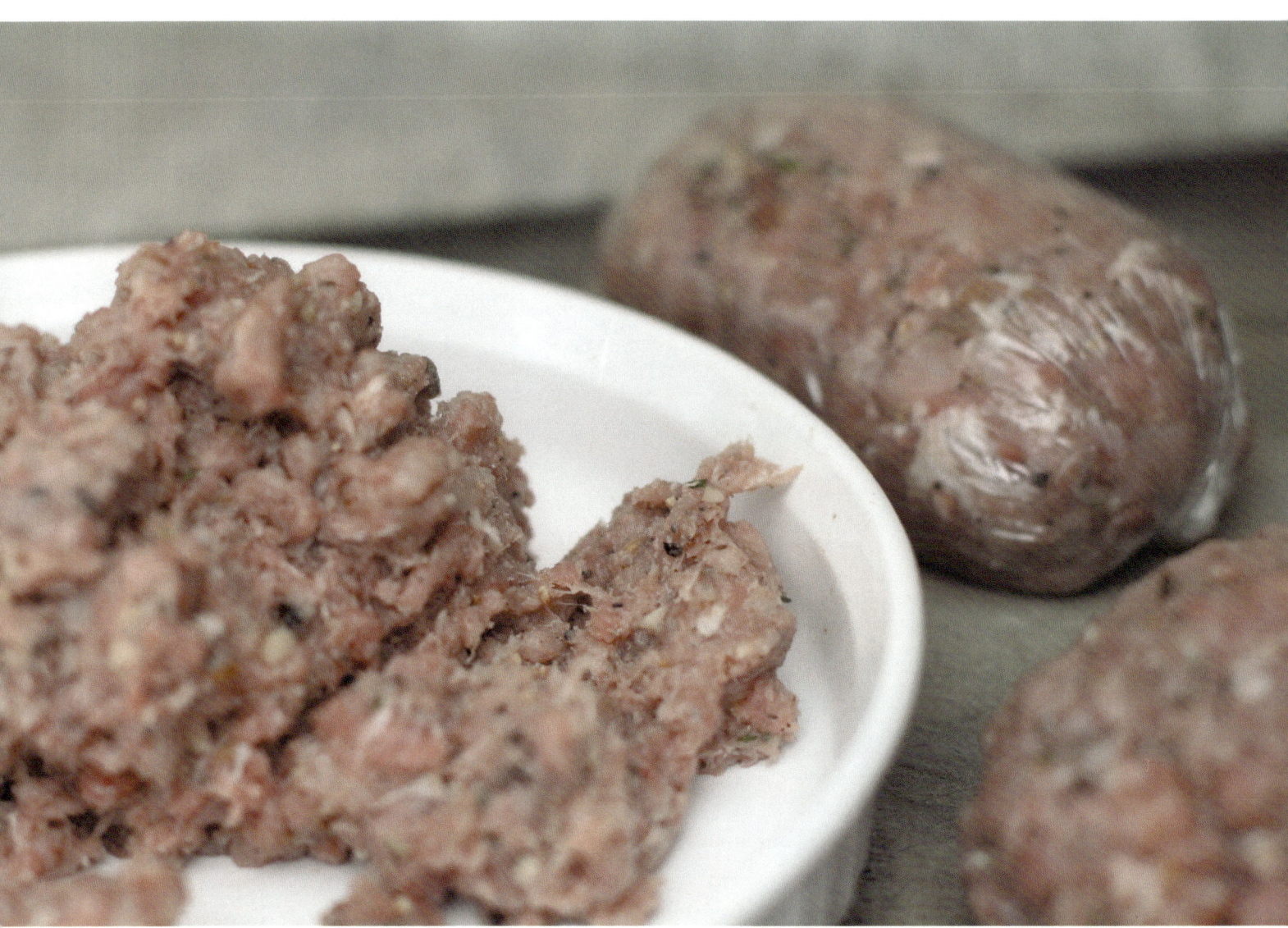

HOMEMADE FRESH ITALIAN PORK SAUSAGE
Salsiccia Fresca

Yields approx. 3 pounds

My mother used to take me to the markets in town; these were usually divided by pavilions, with fruits and vegetables, grains, flowers, and live poultry and meat. The aroma of freshly cut meat, sausages, and salted dry cured meats could be smelled from afar.

Pork is very popular in countries throughout Europe, including Spain, Portugal, and Italy. During the 16th century Inquisition, a lack of pork in the kitchen was seen as evidence of a person having not converted to Catholicism.

Lower-grade cuts of meats and a lot of fat are ground to make the sausages; for that reason, we now make our own, using only fresh herbs, spices, and leftover red wine to marinate the meat; no additives, artificial colorings, or chemicals are needed.

Ingredients

1 tablespoon of fennel seeds, lightly toasted

1 tablespoon of fresh chopped garlic

1 tablespoon of fresh rosemary or fresh sage

1 tablespoon of freshly ground pepper

1 tablespoon of sea salt

2 tablespoons of olive oil

3 pounds pork loin, trimmed of excess fat and cut into two-inch cubes

1 cup of red wine

In a small pan, toast the fennel seeds; remove from heat and lightly crush.

In a large ceramic bowl, mix the rest of the ingredients, cover, and let it marinate in the fridge overnight.

Using a food processor, ground the meat to a coarse consistency; it can be used right away, or formed into rolls, covered with plastic wrap, and frozen for later use.

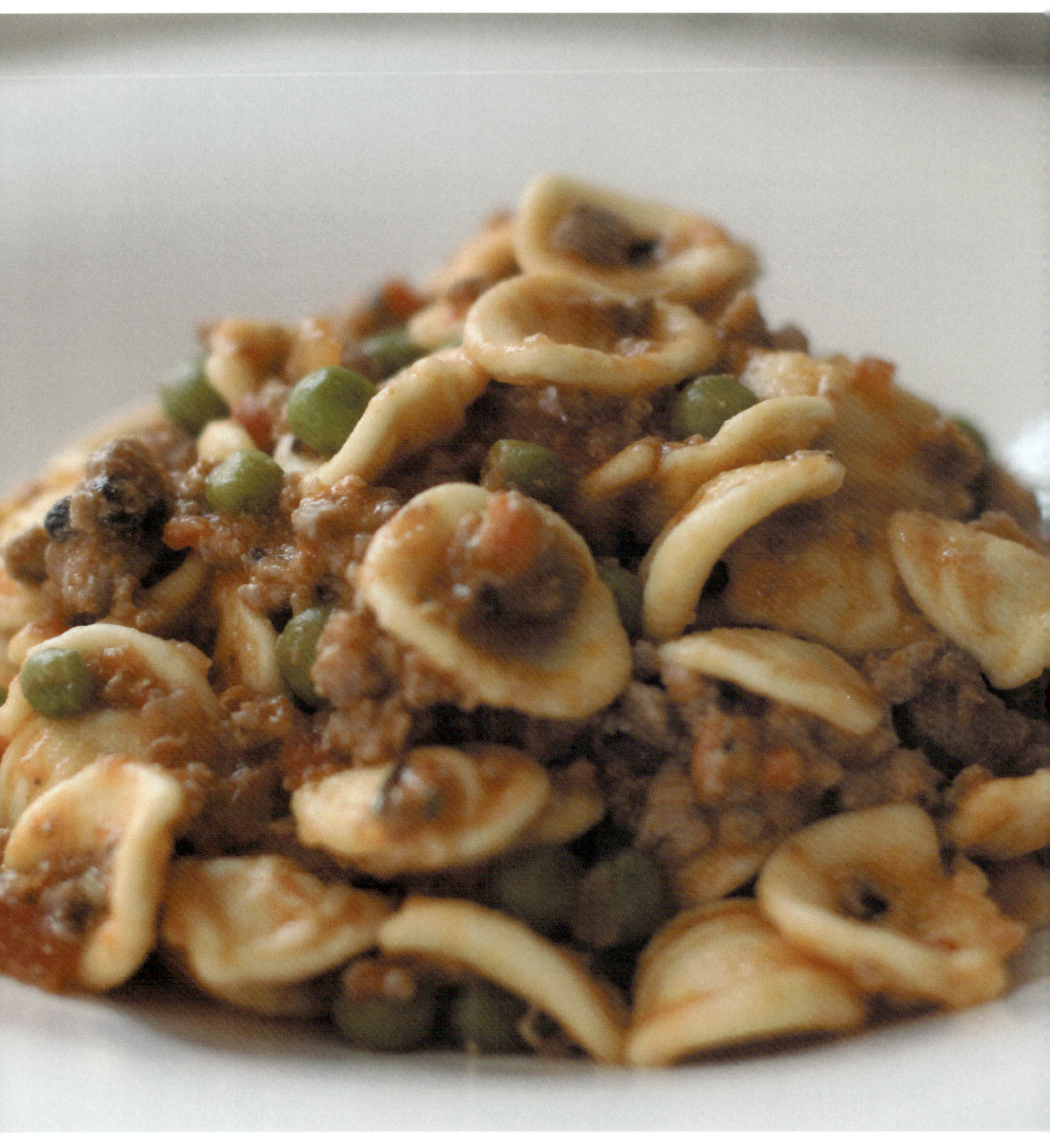

PASTA WITH CREAMY SAUSAGE, PEAS TOMATO SAUCE

Pasta con Salsa di Pomodoro con Panna, Salsiccia e Piseli

Serves 4

We love to explore the surrounding areas in and around New York City. One of our favorite weekend destinations is Cold Spring, located on the east bank of the beautiful Hudson River; it's filled with antique shops, nineteenth-century architecture, and has restaurants and awesome views of the mountains. Our favorite restaurant is Cathryn's Tuscan Grill, which has a beautiful front garden patio where you can sit and have a leisurely late lunch or dinner.

Among the choices on their menu is pasta with a creamy sausage sauce—a very straightforward recipe with amazing flavor. Determined to recreate a similar dish at home, we used our own sausage to limit the amount of fat; you can also use a good quality sweet Italian sausage, with or without fennel, from the store.

This is a great all-in-one dinner, and can be prepared in about half an hour.

Ingredients

3 tablespoons extra virgin olive oil

1–1½ pounds of sweet Italian sausage (with or without fennel) with casings removed; or, follow the recipe for Homemade Fresh Italian Pork Sausage on page 127.)

1 medium-size onion, finely chopped

1 tablespoon fresh sage, finely chopped

1 cup crushed Italian tomatoes

1 cup heavy cream

1 cup (frozen) peas

1 cup of water, added incrementally to adjust thickness of sauce

Orecchiete, farfalle, or your favorite type of pasta, enough for the number of people you are serving. We usually measure 1½ cups of dry or fresh pasta per person.

Chopped parsley for garnish

Fill a large pot with water and set it on the stove over high heat; bring to a boil.

In a separate large pot, heat the olive oil at medium-high heat; add the sausage and break into very small pieces with a wooden spoon; cook for about 15 minutes. Add the onion and sage and cook until the onion is translucent.

Add the tomato and cook until the juice of the tomatoes has evaporated. Add the cream and some water from the sauce and cook for about 10 minutes. Next, add the peas and continue cooking for 10 minutes.

Adjust the thickness of the sauce to your own preference by adding or omitting water. Remove from heat and set aside, covered.

Add salt to the boiling water and cook your pasta as directed on the box; drain when cooked and serve with the sauce. Garnish with chopped parsley.

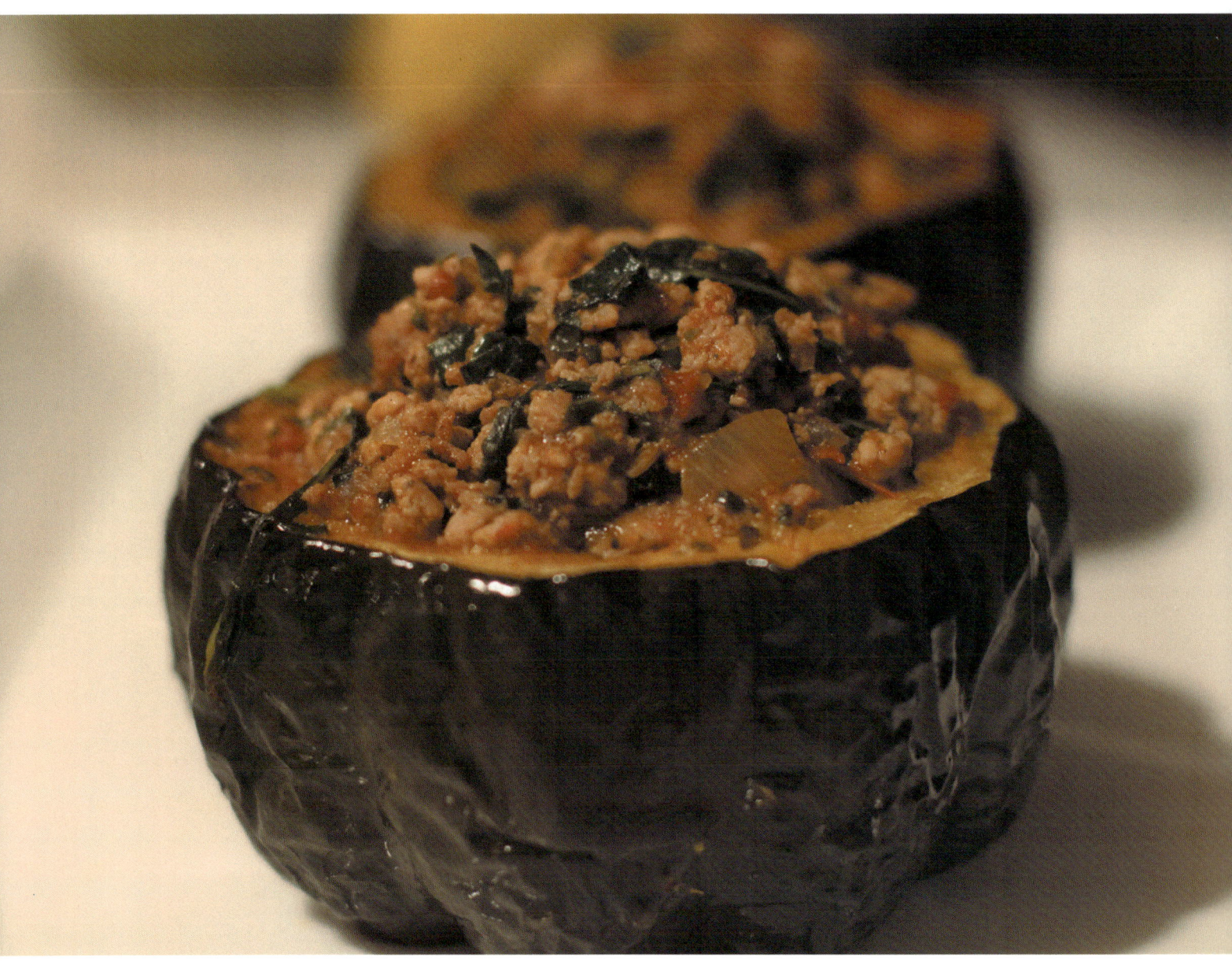

I have always had a fascination with squashes since I was very young; I can recall going to the market with my mother or grandmother to buy pumpkins, but not for decoration—that would have been sacrilegious. I'd gaze at the dozens of shapes, sizes, and colors, just as I did when studying cooking in Italy. They had beautiful names: Delica, Napoletana, Violino, Cappello del prete, Piacentina, among others.

At home they would be turned into so many delicious dishes, and barely anything went to waste. My job was to clean the seeds of any pulp and lay them out under the sun; they would later become toasted snacks or would be ground to make a sauce based on a centuries-old recipe.

ACORN SQUASH STUFFED WITH SAUSAGE AND BLACK KALE

Zucca Ripiene con Salciccia e Cavolo Nero

Serves 2

Buttercup squash is very common through-out northern Italy, where it is known as Delica. Here, turned into a savory dish, the sweet roasted flesh of the squash is a deli-cious contrast to the sausage and black kale filling. You can substitute Buttercup with Acorn squash.

Ingredients

2 medium-size buttercup squash,
    top cut, seeded

Sea salt

Freshly ground black pepper

2 tablespoons extra virgin olive oil

4–5 sweet Italian sausages, casings removed

1 large yellow onion, finely chopped

1 cloves garlic, finely chopped

1 tablespoon fresh sage

2 cups (tightly packed) chopped black kale

2 cups chicken broth

3 tablespoons plain breadcrumbs

¼ cup grated Parmesan cheese plus 2
    tablespoons, divided

Pre-heat oven to 375°F.

Cut the top off of the squash to create a bowl, spoon the seeds and pulp out, and scrape some of the flesh; reserve the flesh, chop it, and set aside.

Sprinkle the squash with salt and pepper; coat with 1 tablespoon of olive oil. Place squash flesh side down on a baking sheet lined with aluminum foil; bake until golden and tender, 30–45 minutes. Remove from oven; flip squash and set aside. Keep the oven on.

In a large skillet over medium heat, heat remaining olive oil. Add sausage; cook, breaking into coarse pieces until brown, 10–15 minutes; you can skim off some of the fat.

Add the onion and the chopped squash flesh to the sausage and cook until soft, about 10 minutes. Add the sage and garlic; cook until the garlic releases its aroma. Add kale and toss; then add broth. Cover and cook until kale is tender. Add the bread crumbs and mix well. Mixture should be moist, not dry. Add one-quarter cup of Parmesan cheese, season-ing with salt and pepper if needed. Remove from heat.

Fill the squash (already on the same baking sheet) with the sausage and kale mixture, sprinkle with the remaining two tablespoons of Parmesan cheese, and bake for about 15–20 minutes or until the cheese on top has melted.

Remove from the oven, serve hot.

DESSERTS

Dolce

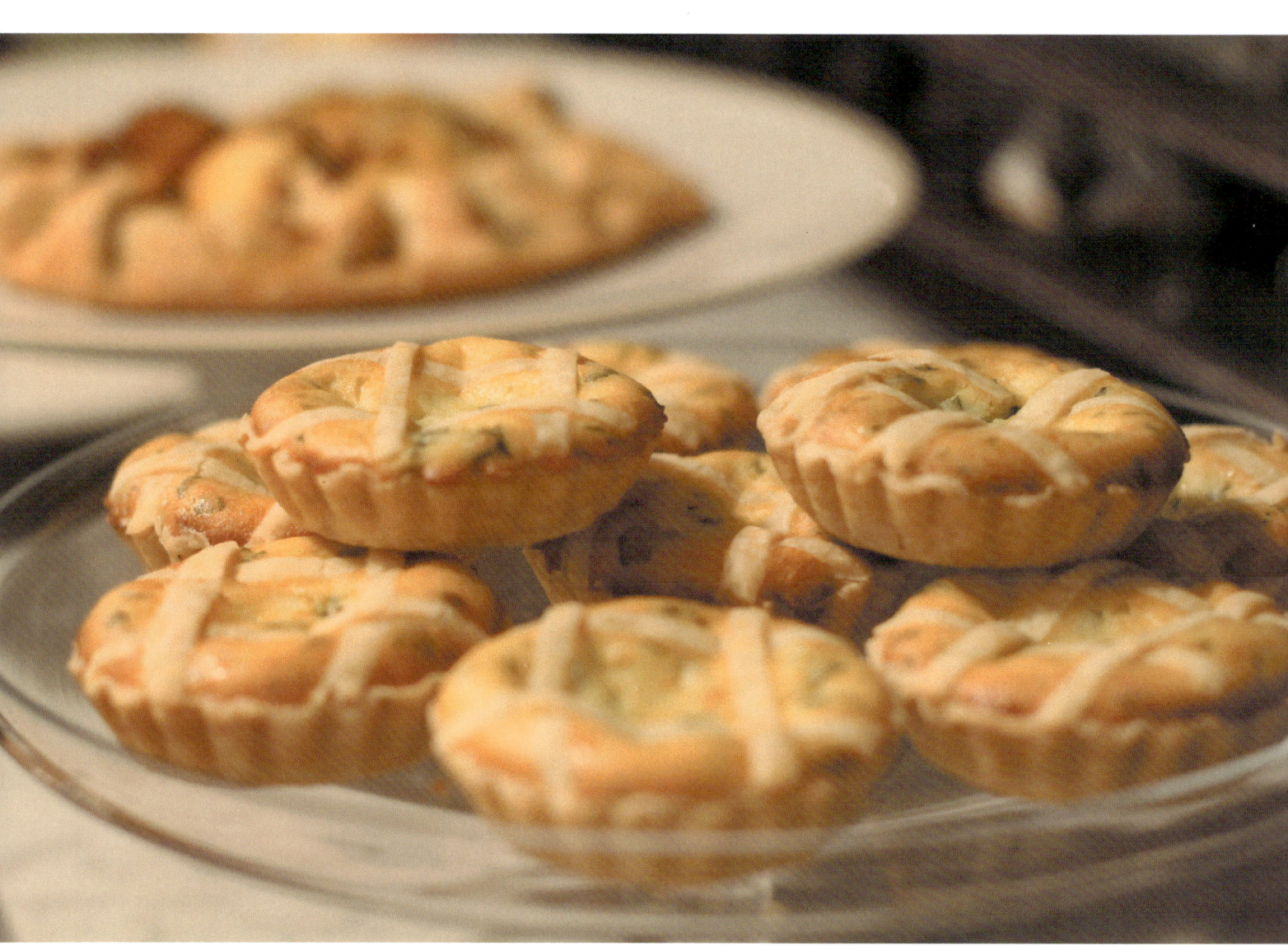

DOLCE RICOTTA TARTLETS WITH FRESH BASIL AND LEMON ZEST

Pasticcini di Ricotta, Basilico e Limone

Serves 12

Basil is not limited to sauces—it's widely used in desserts such as panna cotta, gelato, and lemonade, and is combined with fresh strawberries. This is a family recipe, using just a few ingredients which results in a wonderfully light savory tartlet. These are as beautiful as they are delicious and only require a short preparation time.

Ingredients

3 cups ricotta cheese

½ cup plus 1 tablespoon granulated sugar

Zest of 8 large lemons, finely chopped

20–25 large basil leaves, finely chopped

½ cup Pillsbury all-purpose bleached flour

2 eggs, lightly beaten

3 Pillsbury pie crusts

Equipment

Large mixing bowl

Whisk

10 nonstick tartlet pans 3 × ¾ inches

Citrus zester

Pre-heat oven to 375°F.

In a large bowl, mix the ricotta and sugar with a whisk; add the lemon zest, basil, and flour until well combined. In a small bowl, beat the egg and add to the ricotta mix until thoroughly combined and turned creamy.

Cut 2 of the pie crust into 10 rounds, slightly larger than the tartlet pans, and line the nonstick tartlets. Cut the remaining pastry dough into strips.

Spoon the ricotta mix into the pie crust and use the remaining dough strips to form a lattice pattern over the filling.

Place the tartlets on a baking sheet and bake for 35–40 minutes. They are done when golden brown. Remove from the oven and cool completely.

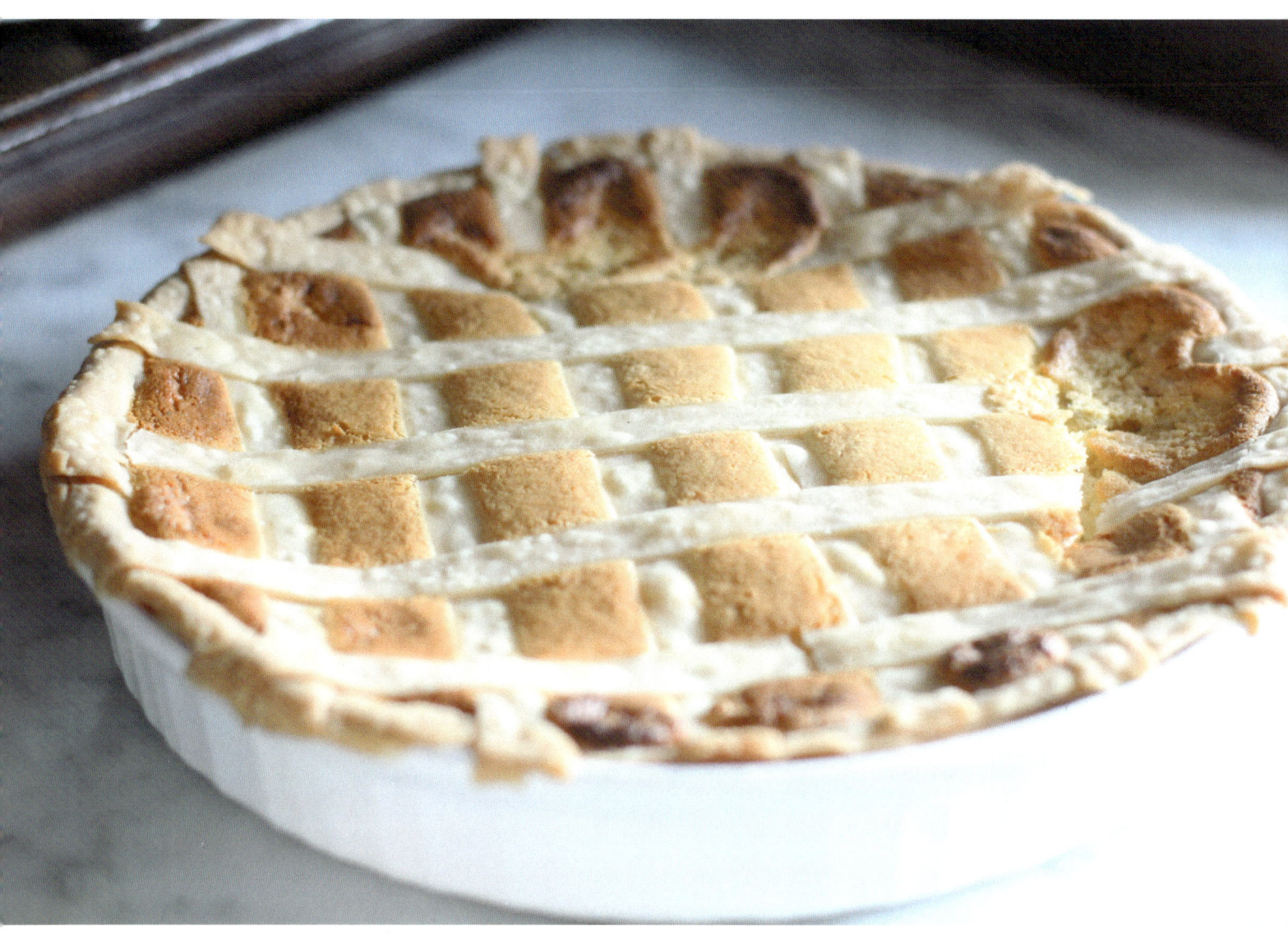

TUSCAN RICOTTA TART

Crostata Di Ricotta Alla Toscana

Serves 8–10

Ricotta means "re-cooked" in Italian. You may think it is a cheese however it is more of a milk product derived by using the watery liquid known as "whey" left over from making cheese. It can be used in so many different ways such as filling for pork, pastas and desserts.

This crostata has the consistency of bread pudding or custard and lacks the heaviness of the standard American Cheese Cake.

Ingredients

½ cup golden raisins

½ cup Marsala wine (sweet) plus 4 tablespoons

4 eggs, separated

¾ cup granulated sugar

½ cup heavy cream

1 teaspoon pure vanilla extract

Grated zest of 4 lemons and juice of 1 lemon

1 tablespoon all-purpose flour plus 1 tablespoon for dusting the pan

2 cups whole milk ricotta

2 ready-made, unrolled pie crust (one is for lattice ribbons half an inch in width)

9 inch pie mold

Put the raisins and half cup of Marsala wine in a bowl and let it soak for 30 minutes.

Next, preheat your oven to 350°F.

Beat the egg yolks and sugar, cream, four tablespoons of Marsala wine, vanilla, and zest until thoroughly combined. Add one tablespoon of flour and mix in the ricotta.

Wash your beaters well, and then beat the egg whites with 1 teaspoon of lemon juice in a separate bowl until stiff peaks form. Gently fold the egg whites into the batter.

Roll out the crust onto a greased pie mold, also lightly dusted with flour, and cut the excess dough.

Spoon the ricotta mix into the piecrust and use the remaining dough to form a lattice pattern over the filling.

Bake for one hour.

Remove the tart form the oven, let it stand for at least 25 minutes.

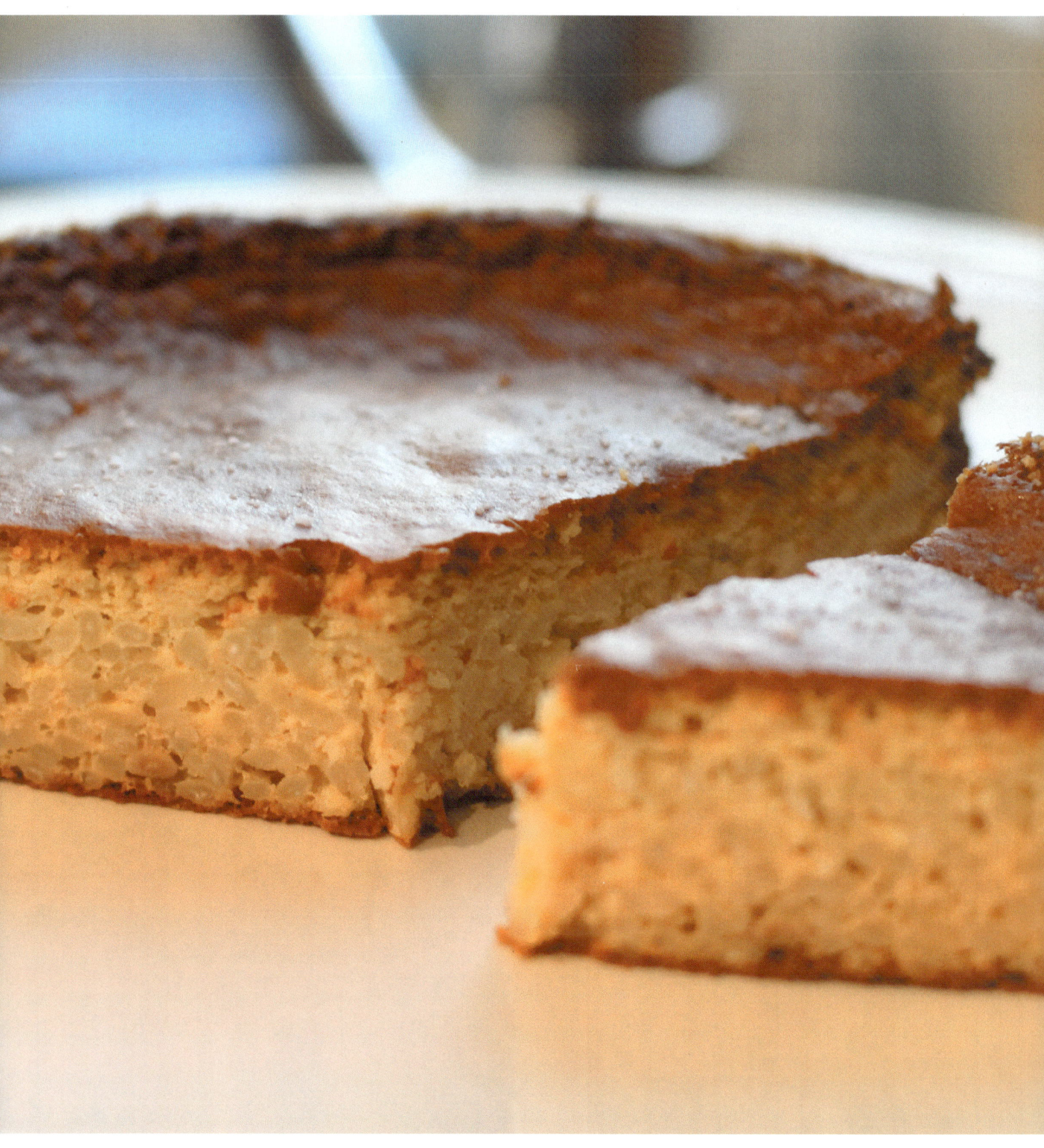

ARBORIO CAKE
Torta degli Addobbi

This cake was usually made only during Easter, particularly in Bologna. In Spain it is known as Budin de Arroz, with a much richer consistency given by the condensed milk and a hint of nutmeg instead of vanilla.

Ingredients

5 cups of milk

⅓ cup Arborio rice

1¼ cups sugar

2 tablespoons extra virgin olive oil

Rind of 3 lemons

1 cup of chopped almonds

4 eggs

2 teaspoons of pure vanilla extract

Plain bread crumbs

Pre-heat the oven to 350°F.

Bring the milk to a boil and add the rice, vanilla extract, sugar, olive oil, and lemon rind.

Cook for 40–45 minutes, until the rice is al dente, then remove from heat and add the almonds. Leave the mixture to cool, stirring occasionally.

In a bowl, beat the eggs and add to the cooled rice, then mix well.

Pour the mixture into a nine-inch baking pan that has been buttered and dusted with the plain breadcrumbs; bake for an hour or until a knife comes out clean from the middle of the cake.

Remove from oven and let it cool completely. Remove from pan and dust with powdered sugar on top.

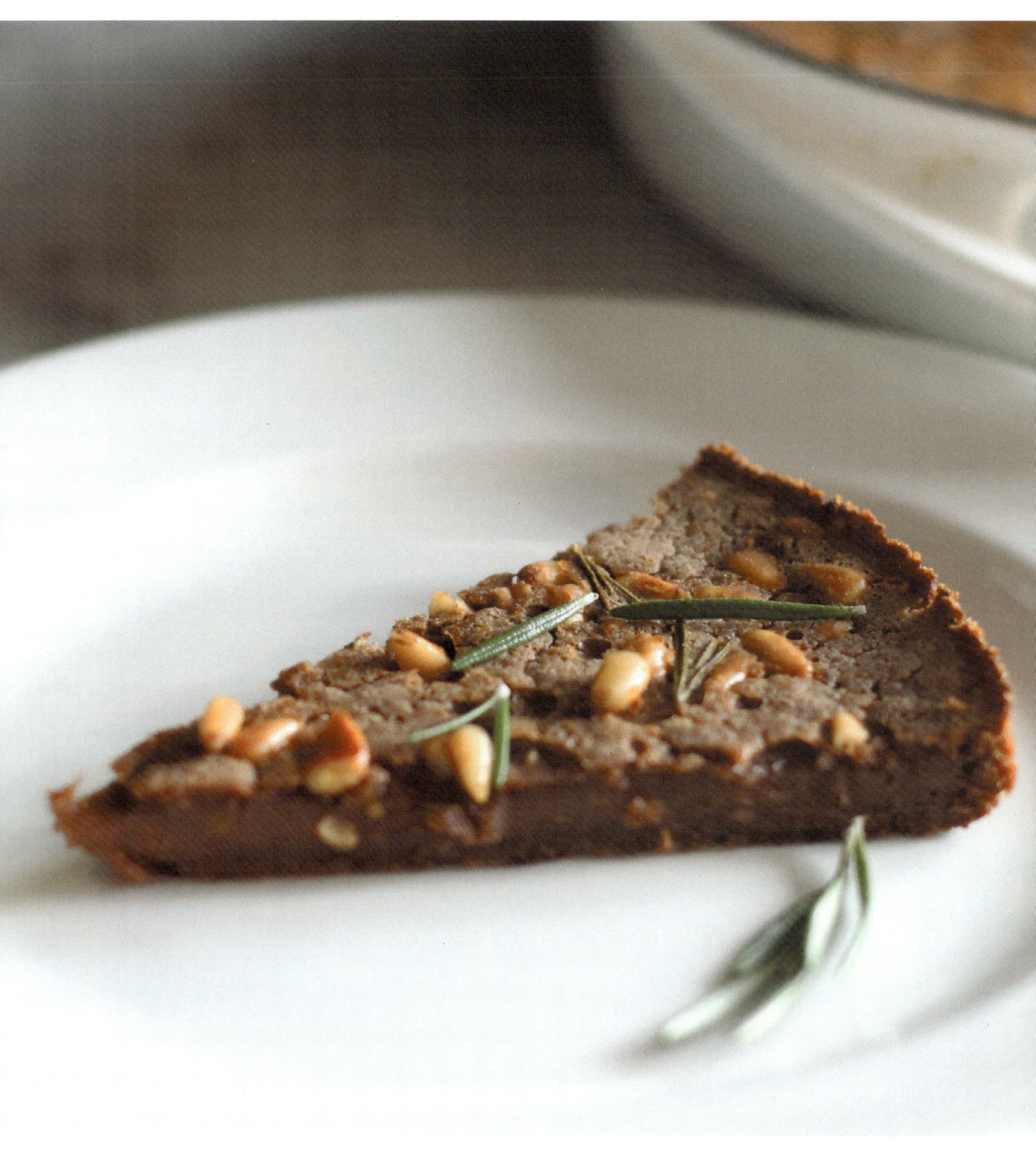

CHESTNUT CAKE
Castagnaccio

Serves 4

"La torta dei uomini poveri."

This is a traditional autumn Tuscan dessert. It has a unique and hearty flavor, almost like a mild chocolate. The fresh rosemary is not just for decoration; it brings an extraordinary, unexpected combination of taste to the natural sweetness of the chestnut flour.

There is no sugar added (or needed) and it's naturally gluten-free!

Ingredients

½ pound chestnut flour

2 cups of cold water

⅓ cup of golden raisins, soaked in warm water for 15–20 minutes.

¼ cup of pine nuts

1 tablespoon or less of fresh rosemary, needles only

Zest of 1 lemon

3 tablespoons of extra virgin olive oil, plus a little extra for drizzling on top

Sea salt, a pinch

Plain bread crumbs for dusting the baking pan

Pre-heat the oven to 375°F.

Oil a nine-inch baking pan and dust with the bread crumbs; shake excess off, set aside.

Drain the raisins that have been soaking in warm water.

In a large bowl, mix the flour, pinch of salt, olive oil, and half of the water; combine well and long enough to eliminate any lumps. Add the lemon zest and remaining water; mixture will be runny, almost like the consistency of crêpe mix.

Pour the mix in the baking pan. Sprinkle the raisins on top of the mixture, then the pine nuts, and last, the rosemary. Drizzle some extra olive oil on top, and bake for 40–45 minutes. The cake will not rise, and is ready when its surface is golden brown and cracked.

Remove from the oven and let it cool completely.

Traditionally served with ricotta, this cake is as just as good served plain.

Chestnut flour is found at specialty stores such as Whole Foods or online gourmet stores.

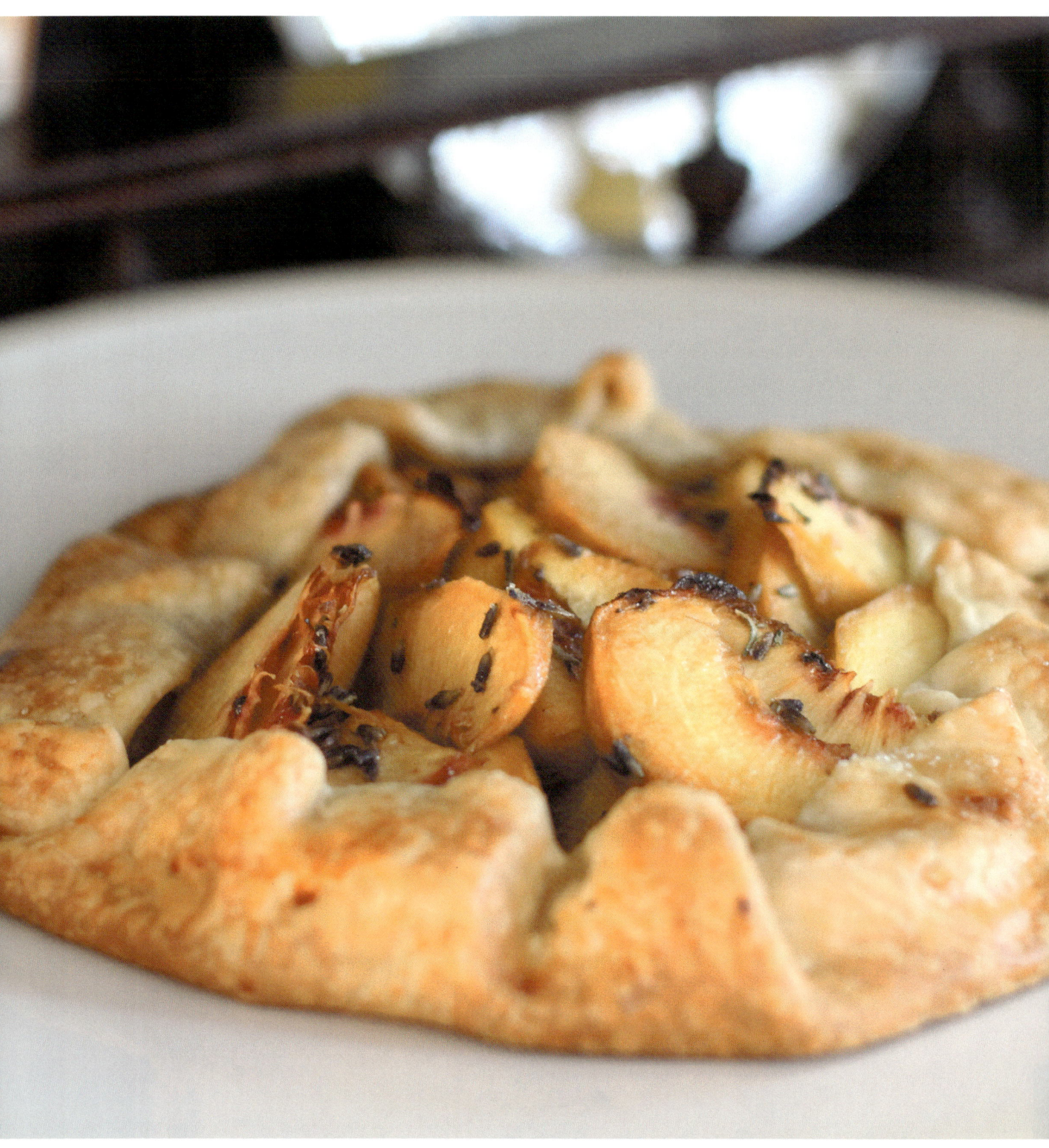

PEACH CROSTATA WITH ROSEMARY AND LAVENDER

Crostata di Pesche, Rosemarino e Lavanda

Serves 6

Lavender doesn't bring Italian cooking to mind, but it has been used since Roman times. This crostata recipe combines lavender and rosemary, creating a surprisingly easy to make and delicious rustic dessert.

Ingredients

1 pre-made refrigerated pie crust, softened as directed on box

For the filling:

3–4 medium-size unpeeled ripe peaches, cut into slices

¼ cup sugar, plus a little extra for the top

1 tablespoon olive oil

1 large sprig each of rosemary and lavender, leaves chopped

1 egg yolk, mixed with a little water (also known as an egg wash)

Preheat the oven to 425°F.

Put all the ingredients above into a mixing bowl and mix them well.

Place the pie crust on a lined baking sheet and pile the peaches in the middle of the round, letting them spread out in a natural way while leaving about a two-inch border all around. If they've given off a lot of juice, leave some of it in the bowl. Fold the edge of the pastry up and around the fruit, pleating the edges as you go. You should have a large opening in the middle where the peaches stick out.

Brush the exposed part of the crust with the egg wash and sprinkle a little sugar all over the tart.

Bake until the crust is golden, about 35 minutes. Let it cool before serving.

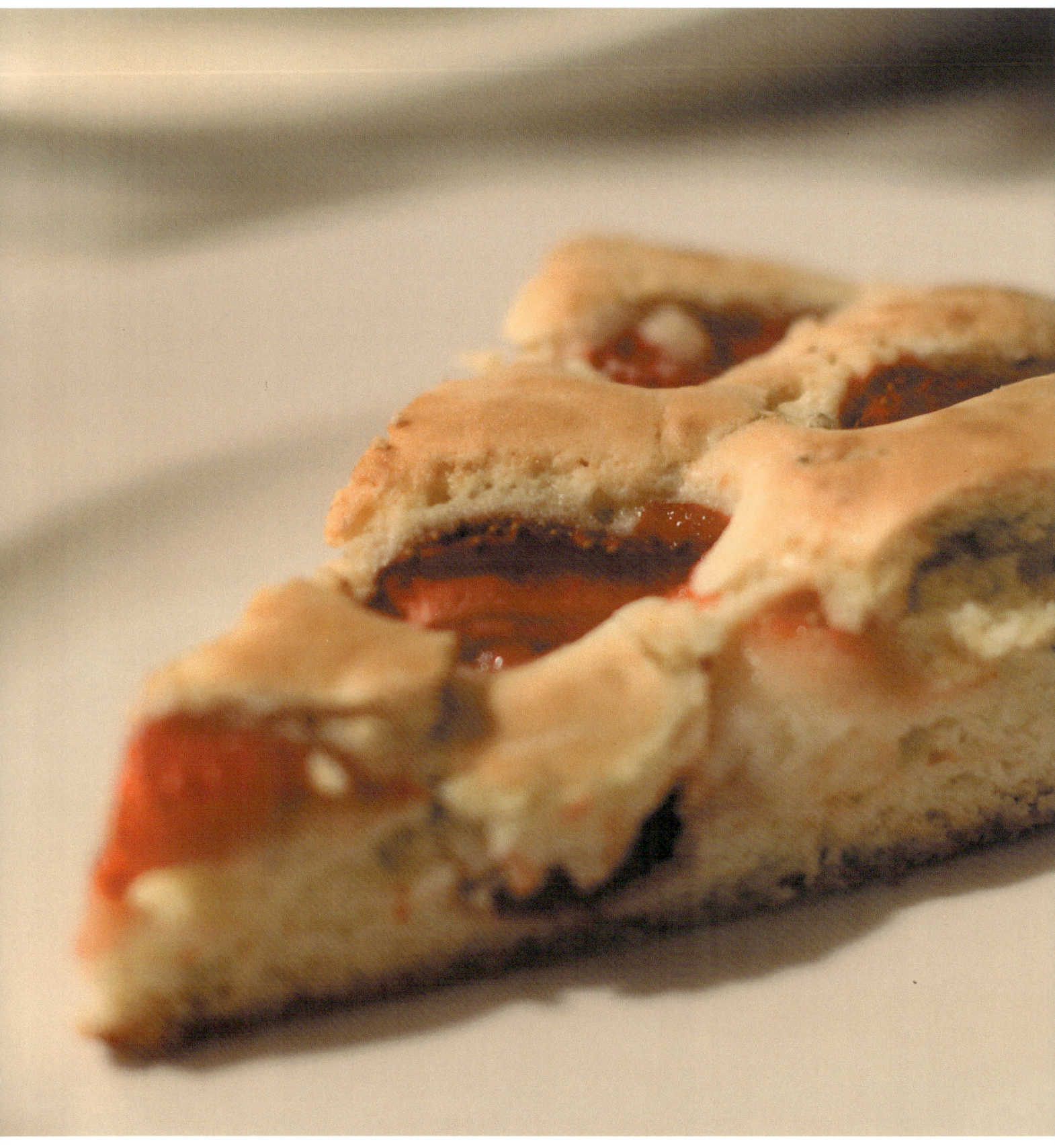

STRAWBERRY, BASIL, AND OLIVE OIL CAKE

Torta di Fragola, Basilico, e Olio d'Oliva

Serves 4-6

This summer cake joins juicy strawberries and fresh basil with the piquancy provided by the olive oil. It is delicious and can serve as a mid-afternoon snack with coffee as well as dessert!

Ingredients

1½ cups all-purpose flour

¼ teaspoon sea salt

1 tablespoon baking powder

2 large eggs

½ cup plus 2 tablespoons of sugar

¾ cup olive oil

⅓ cup milk

⅓ cup dry Marsala wine or Madeira, Port or Pinot Noir

½ cup fresh basil, finely chopped

Zest of 1 lemon

1 cup fresh strawberries, sliced in halves

Confectioner's sugar for decoration (optional)

9 or 10 inch round springform pan

Preheat oven to 375°F.

In a bowl, mix the flour, salt, and baking powder.

Using an electric mixer, combine the eggs and sugar and beat until it becomes creamy.

Gradually add the olive oil, milk, wine, lemon zest and basil.

Lower the speed and add the flour mix until thoroughly combined.

Grease and lightly flour the baking pan; pour the batter into the pan and place the strawberries on top of the batter all around. Bake on the middle rack for about 45–50 minutes. Check for doneness when a knife comes out clean from the center of the cake.

Let it cool completely and dust with powdered sugar.

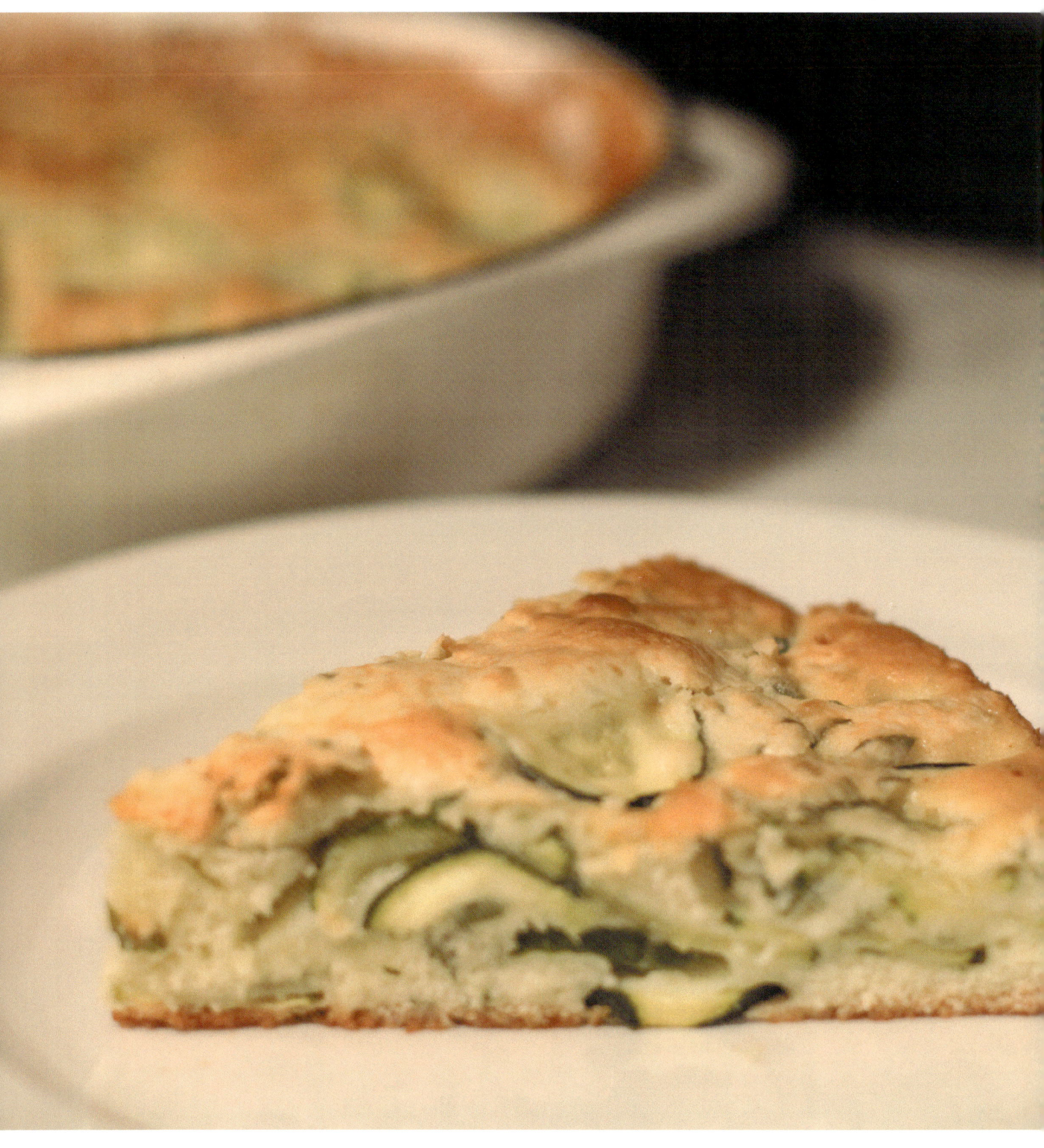

ZUCCHINI AND BASIL CAKE
Scarpaccia

Serves 4-6

This is a typical peasant dessert from the town of Viareggio, north of Pisa. A wholesome sweet cake made with extra virgin olive oil, zucchini, and fresh basil.

Ingredients

Olive oil and plain bread crumbs to dust the baking pan

2 large eggs

1½ cup sugar

¼ cup extra virgin olive oil

A pinch of sea salt

8–10 medium-size basil leaves, minced

3 medium-size zucchini, slightly over one pound, thinly sliced crosswise

1⅓ cups all-purpose flour

Preheat oven to 375°F.

Lightly oil a nine- or ten-inch round baking pan, dust it with plain bread crumbs, and shake off the excess.

In a large bowl or mixer, beat the eggs and sugar; add olive oil, sea salt, and basil until thoroughly combined. Add the flour and combine well making sure there are no lumps. Add the sliced zucchini and mix well without overdoing it. Pour into the baking pan and even up the top with a spatula or back of a spoon.

Bake for 40–45 minutes. At this point a knife inserted in the center should come out clean.

Let it cool completely, cut into wedges, and serve.

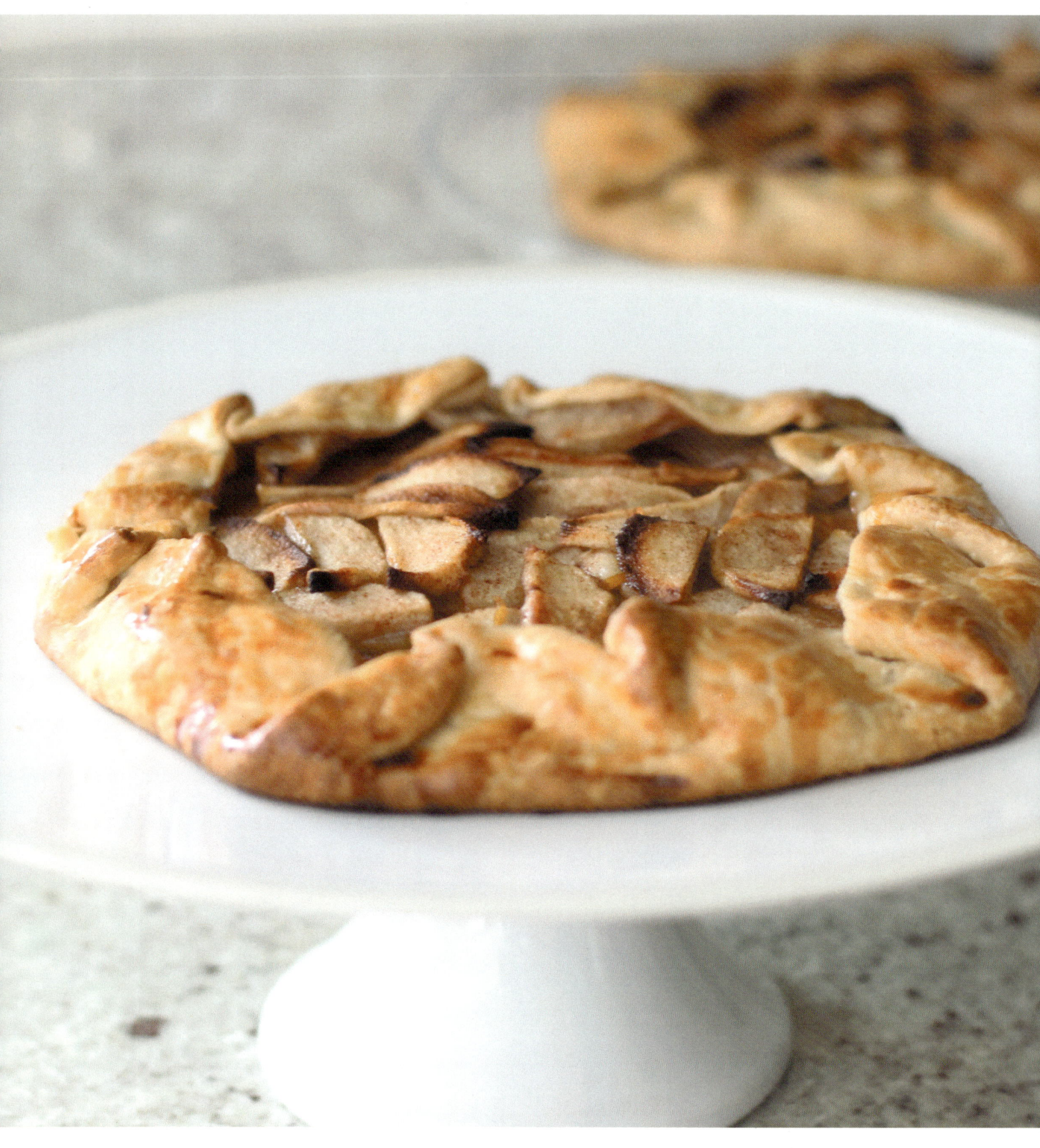

APPLE CROSTATA

Crostata di Mele

Serves 4

This used to be one of the many mid-after-noon snacks Nonna Maria would surprise me with while I studied outside Florence. It was simple and delicious, sometimes flavored with the fresh rosemary that she grew in the garden. Nonna used to say this was her version of American pie.

Ingredients

2 pounds Granny Smith apples, peeled, cored, and cut into quarter-inch slices (4–5)

½ cup granulated sugar

1 teaspoon ground cinnamon

½ teaspoon nutmeg

1 tablespoon all-purpose flour

1 tablespoon extra virgin olive oil

1 teaspoon freshly squeezed lemon juice

1 pre-made pie crust

1 egg yolk mixed with a spoon of cold water (also known as an egg wash)

1 tablespoon granulated sugar

Pre-heat oven to 420°F.

In a large bowl, mix the apples, sugar, cinnamon, nutmeg, flour, olive oil, and lemon juice until the apples are evenly coated. Set aside for 15 minutes.

Unfold the crust on a baking sheet lined with parchment or waxed paper. Arrange the apples in the center, leaving a two- to three-inch border. Fold the dough edges over the apples loosely, leaving the crostata open in the center. Do not pour all the excess liquid from the apples onto the dough as you run the risk of making it soggy. Brush the dough with the egg mixture and sprinkle the tablespoon of sugar on top of the crostata. Bake for 40–45 minutes. By then it should be golden brown.

Remove from oven and let it cool.

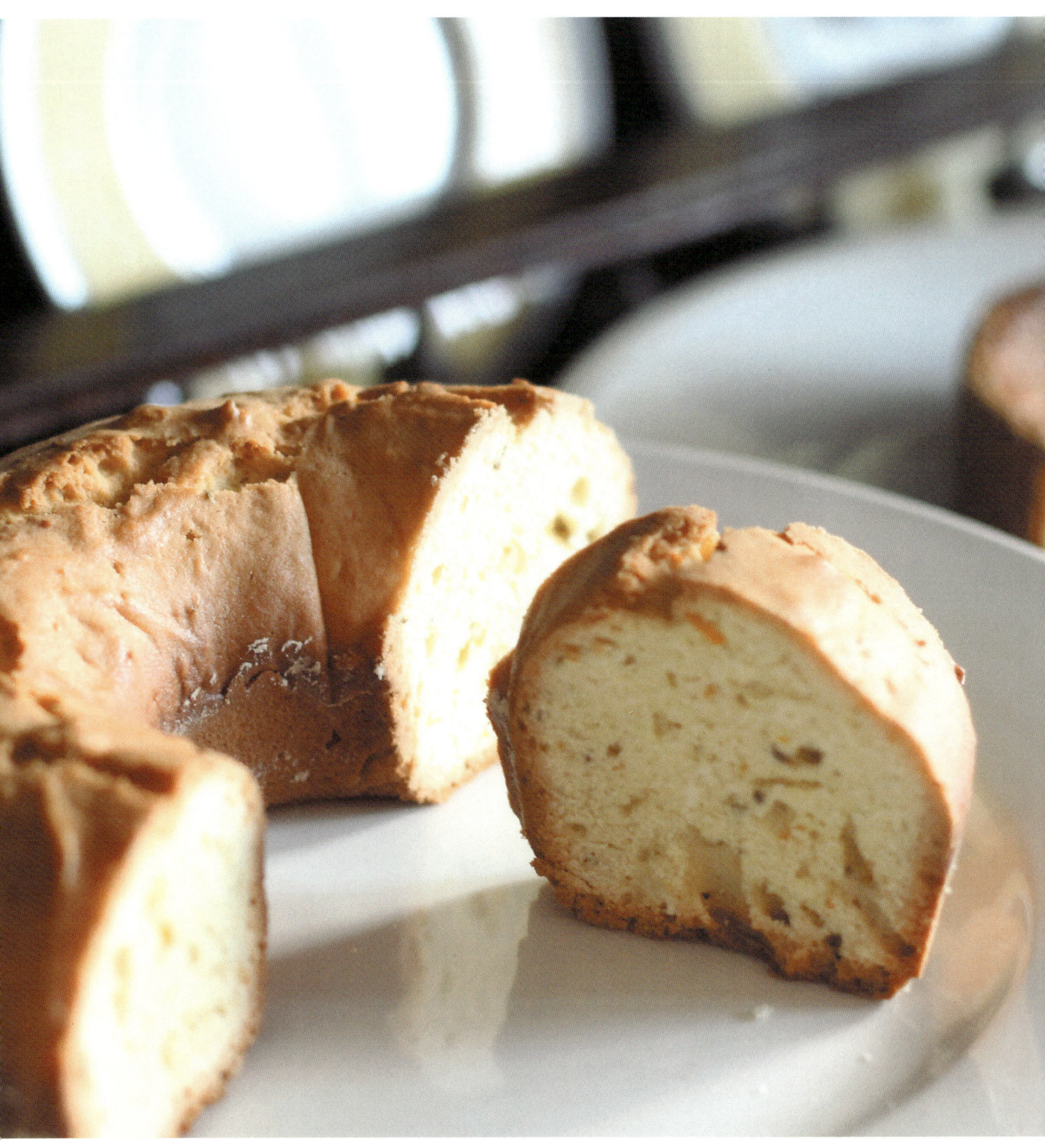

TUSCAN RING CAKE
Ciambellone

Serves 6-8

The Ciambella is one of the most widespread Italian recipes. This term originally refers to sweet ring-shaped bread, and is either baked or fried. Since Ciambella is a generic term, you can find it in different forms, such as cookies and doughnuts, in almost every region in Italy.

My teacher in Florence used to bake hers using a Lavazza coffee can in the middle to form the hole. The classic shape of a ciambella is a ring; in fact, there is an Italian saying when something goes wrong: *Non tutte le ciambelle riescono col buco*, which means, "Not all ciambelle come out with a hole." This is very simple to make and is excellent with a cup of coffee.

Ingredients

5 cups of all-purpose flour (we prefer the Italian "00")

⅛ teaspoon of sea salt

1½ teaspoons of baking powder

5 large eggs

2⅓ cups sugar

¾ cup extra virgin olive oil

1 cup whole milk

Grated zest of two lemons

¼ cup of Limoncello liqueur (optional)

Pre-heat the oven to 385°F.

Lightly butter and flour a twelve-inch ring mold (also known as an angel food cake mold).

In a large bowl, combine the flour, salt, and baking powder, and set aside.

In a large bowl or electric mixer, beat the eggs and sugar until creamy. Stir in the olive oil, milk, lemon zest, and Limoncello (optional). Mix well and slowly incorporate with the flour, salt, and baking powder mixture. Mix until well combined.

Pour the batter into the prepared mold and bake for 50–55 minutes or until a thin knife comes out clean from the center of the cake. The cake at this point should be a beautiful golden brown.

Let it cool completely before serving.

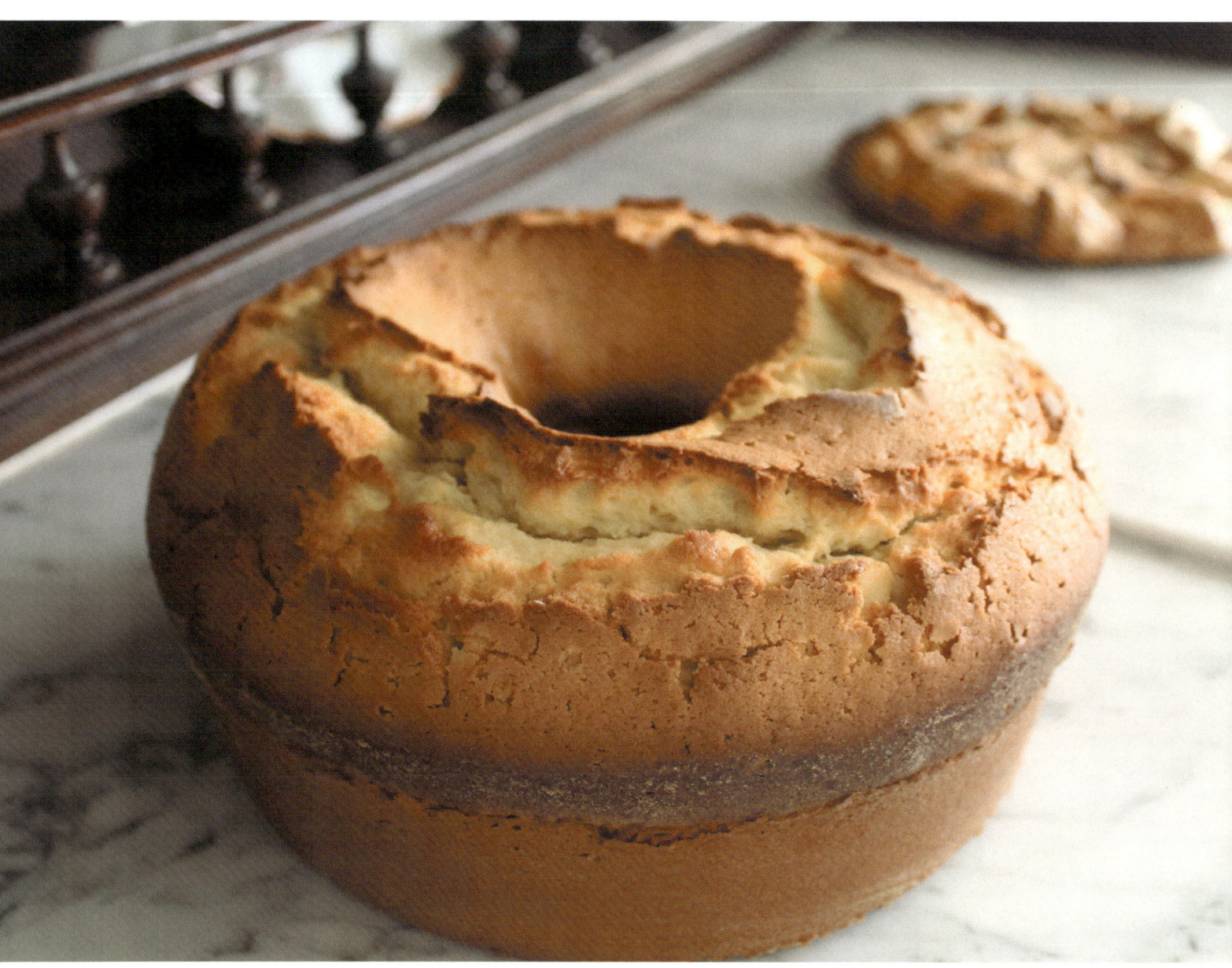

FAT THURSDAY TUSCAN CARNIVALE CAKE
Berlingozzo

Serves 6-8

Berlingozzo is very similar to Ciambellone. The recipe for Berlingozzo calls for ingredients forbidden during the observance of Lent (milk, eggs, and butter). Its name comes from a Tuscan word with German origins: *berlingaccio*, which means "Fat Thursday". The Berlingozzo is traditionally prepared during Carnival, specifically on Fat Thursday. Good for breakfast or a mid-afternoon coffee break.

Ingredients

3 eggs

1 cup sugar

½ cup butter, at room temperature

3 cups all-purpose flour

1½ teaspoons baking powder

Pinch of salt

Grated zest of 2 oranges or 3 lemons

1½ teaspoon of aniseed

Whole milk, 2–3 tablespoons

Pre-heat oven to 350°F. Butter and coat in flour a ring-shaped mold. Beat the eggs with the sugar with a whisk or electric mixer until they become very creamy. Add the butter and continue mixing, then add the flour, baking powder, salt, orange zest, and aniseed until just combined. If the mixture is too thick, add some milk—a couple of tablespoons or more—to obtain a thick but soft and creamy mixture.

Bake for around 30–40 minutes or until risen and golden brown; a knife should come out clean when inserted in the middle of the cake.

Remove from the oven and let it cool completely before cutting.

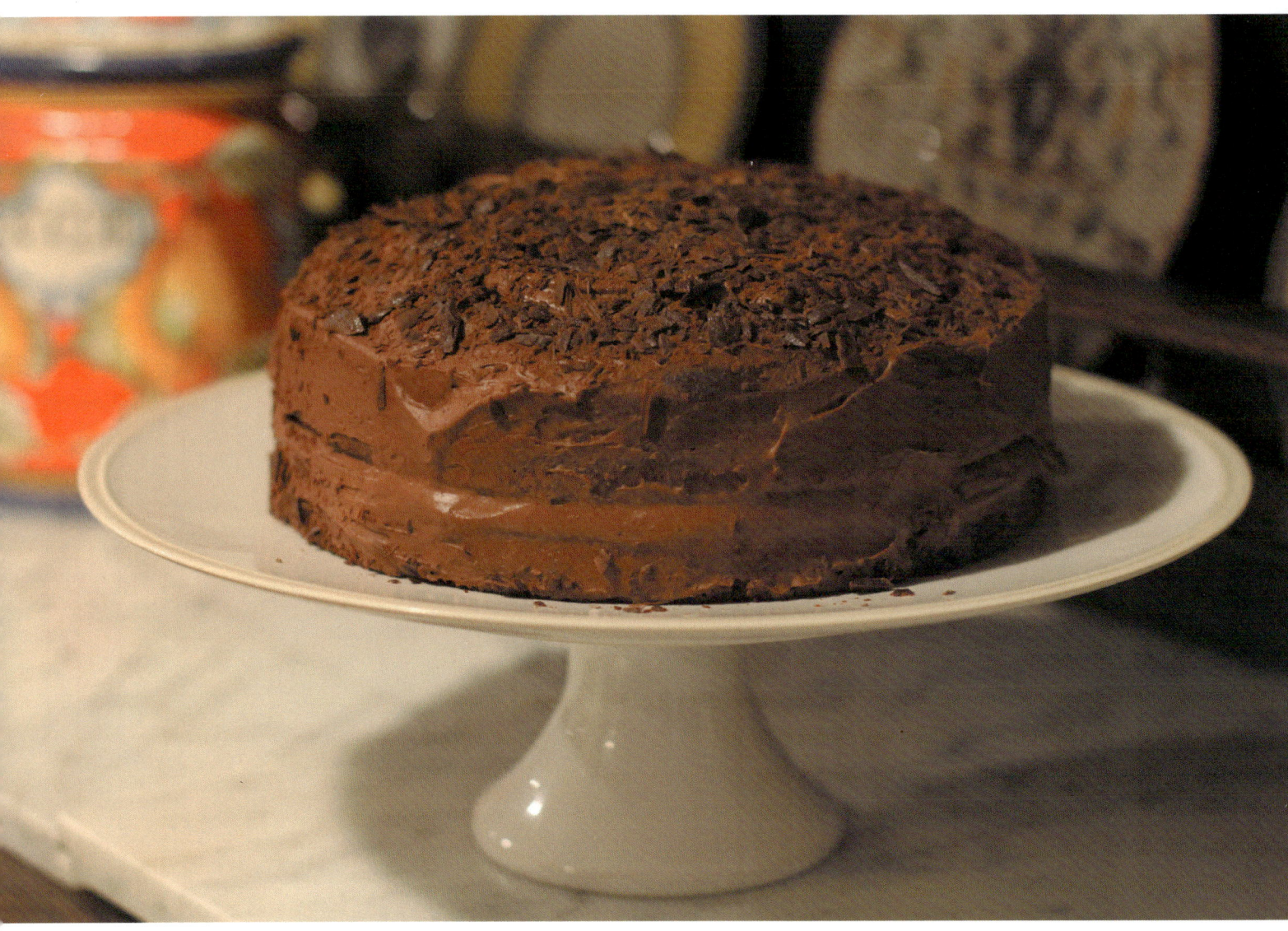

Wine was always an integral part of our daily meals since early childhood. No wine was wasted. Low quality or stale wine was turned into sangria and added to stews or whatever else was cooking.

That nothing-goes-to-waste mentality applies to this easy-to-make cake; any leftover red wine that is still good to drink can go into making this moist and delicious cake. The olive oil adds a yet another layer of piquance to the chocolate and red wine combination.

A favorite in our house, and often requested by family members, it can be made with or without the chocolate mousse as shown in this picture.

CHOCOLATE CAKE WITH OLIVE OIL AND RED WINE

Torta al Cioccolato con Vino Rosso

Ingredients

For the wet mixture:

3 eggs

1¾ cups sugar

1 cup buttermilk *or* watered down sour cream (mix ½ cup of sour cream with ½ cup of cold water)

1 cup red wine such as Chianti, Cabernet Sauvignon, or Shiraz

½ cup plus 2 tablespoons of olive oil

1½ tablespoon pure vanilla extract

For the dry mixture:

2 cups all-purpose flour

1 cup plus 2 tablespoons unsweetened dark cocoa

2 teaspoons baking soda

1 teaspoon baking powder

1 tablespoon of cinnamon

1 teaspoon of salt

Pre-heat the oven to 375°F.

Lightly grease and flour two nine-inch springform pans if you are making it with a chocolate mousse, or a ten-inch Bundt pan if you are making it without it

For the dry mixture: In one bowl, combine the flour, cocoa, baking soda, cinnamon, baking powder, and salt; mix well and set aside.

For the wet mixture: In an electric mixer, beat the eggs with the sugar until creamy; slowly add the buttermilk, wine, olive oil, and vanilla.

At a slow speed, gradually add the dry mix until thoroughly combined, ensuring no lumps of flour have formed. Pour the batter into your prepared pans and bake for about 35 minutes, or until a cake tester inserted into the center comes out clean. Let it cool completely.

Mousse-covered option with two nine-inch cakes:

Chocolate mousse ingredients:

2 cups heavy cream, very cold

1¼ cup dark cocoa powder

1¼ cup powdered sugar

1 teaspoon cinnamon

In a standing mixer fitted with the whip attachment, pour the heavy cream, then add the cocoa powder, cinnamon, and sugar. On low speed, begin to mix the mousse. Start on low or you will be wearing the cocoa powder!

Whip the cream until powder starts to incorporate, stopping occasionally to scrape down the sides. Increase speed to high. Whip the mousse until stiff. Time may vary, about 2–5 minutes, just until stiff.

When the two nine-inch cakes are cool, cover the top of the first one with some of the mousse; place the second one on top and continue to cover completely.

Optional: Decorate the cake with chocolate shavings using a vegetable peeler.

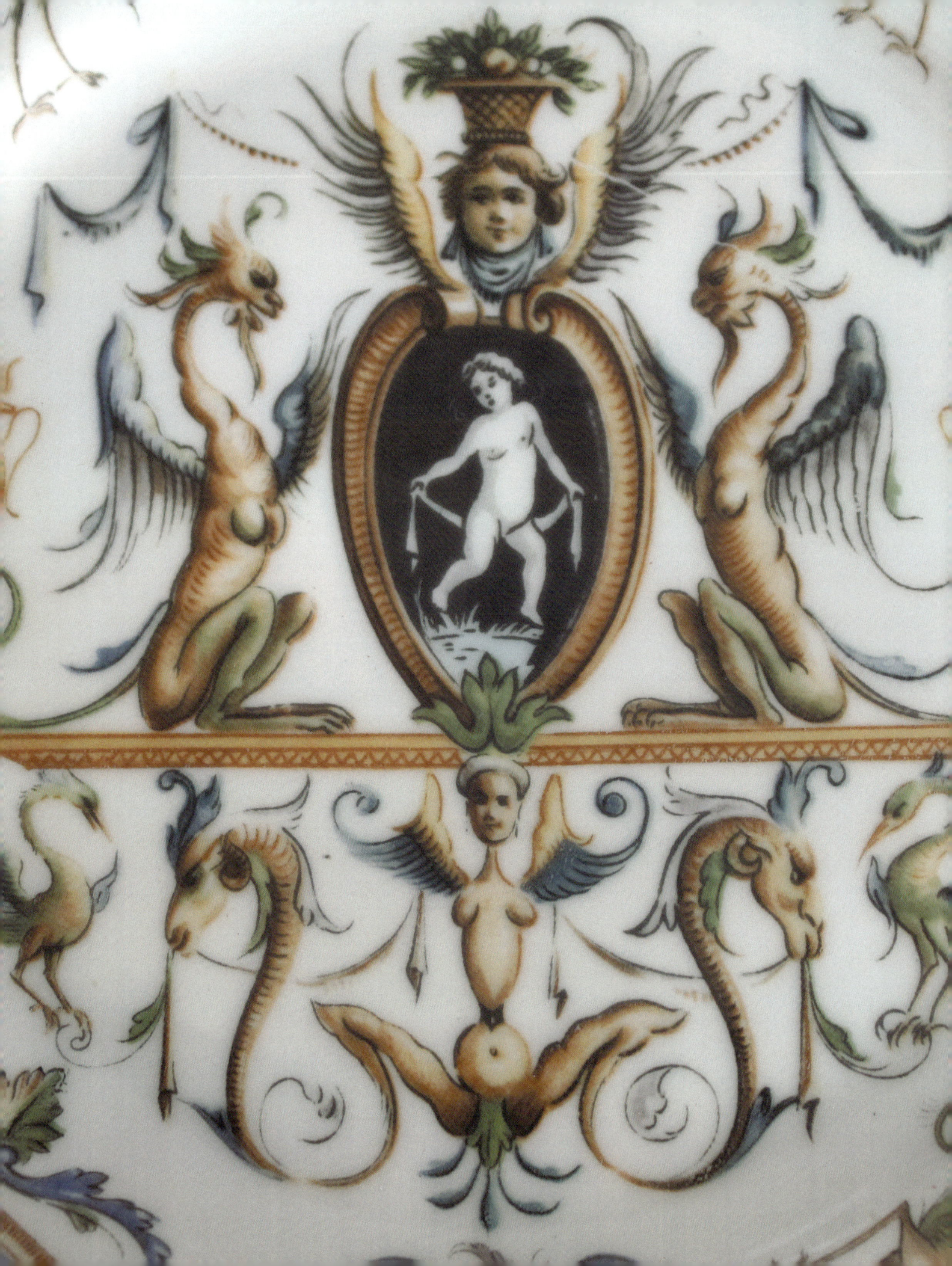

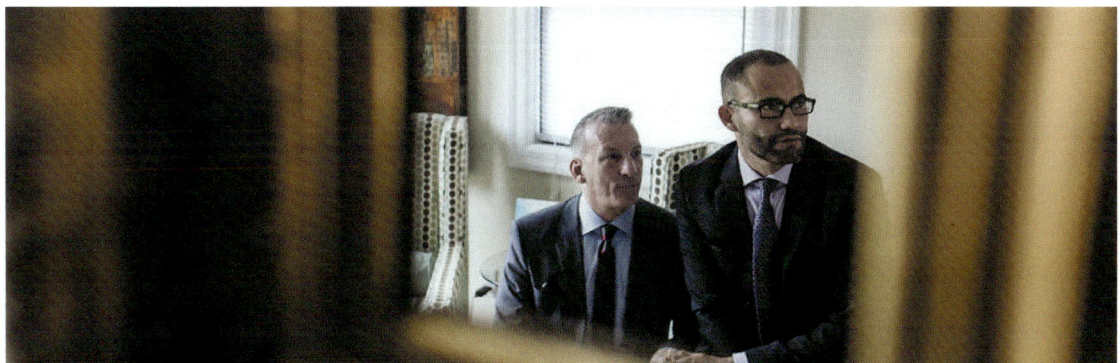

ABOUT THE AUTHORS

From his early teen years, Robert Gray nurtured a dream of writing while Luis Somoza, a lover of food and cooking, honed his culinary expertise from childhood to adulthood. Having grown up with strong maternal role models, both men have been steeped in the joy of celebrating good food, high quality wine, and closeness with family. They live in New York, one of the world's most sophisticated and diverse food capitals, and enjoy extending their hospitality to their friends and loved ones.

CPSIA information can be obtained at www.ICGtesting.com
Printed in the USA
LVIW01n1054230216
476289LV00003B/3